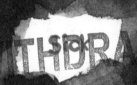

Sick ©2016 Gabby Schulz
Published by Secret Acres
Designed by Gabby Schulz & Leon Avelino

Secret Acres
237 Flatbush Ave. #331
Brooklyn, NY 11217

PCN: 2013956599
ISBN: 978-0-9962739-1-6

SA030

Printed in Hong Kong

A previous version of *Sick* appeared as a serialized
webcomic on gabbysplayhouse.com. It was redrawn
and reprinted by request of Secret Acres.

for Ernestine

He putteth his mouth in the dust; if so be there may be hope.

~ Lamentations 3:29

I did not get my Spaghetti-Os. I got spaghetti.
I want the press to know this.

~ Thomas J. Grasso,
at his execution,
March 20, 1995

ONCE, I GOT SICK.

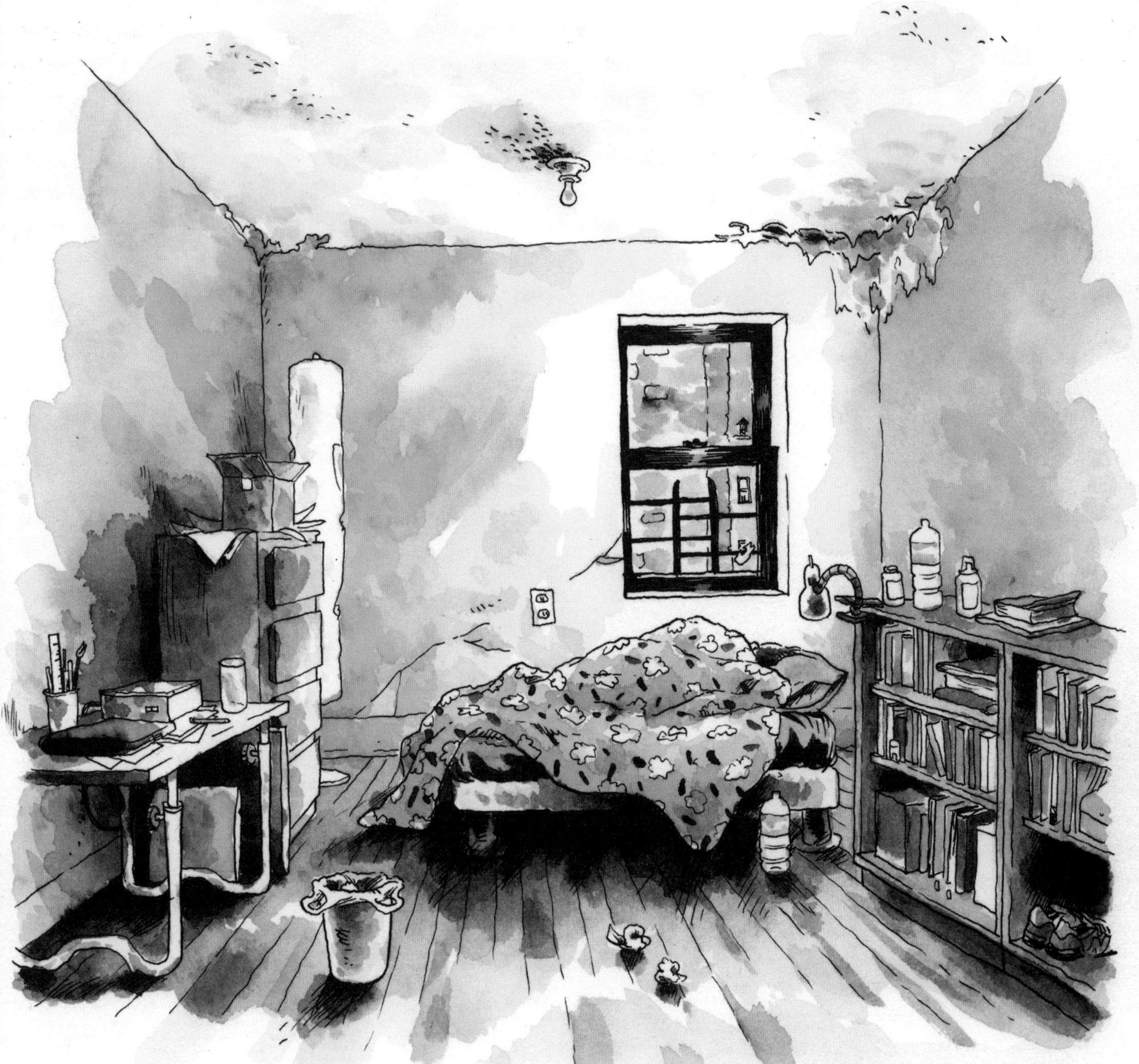

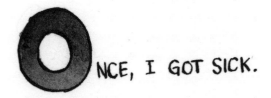

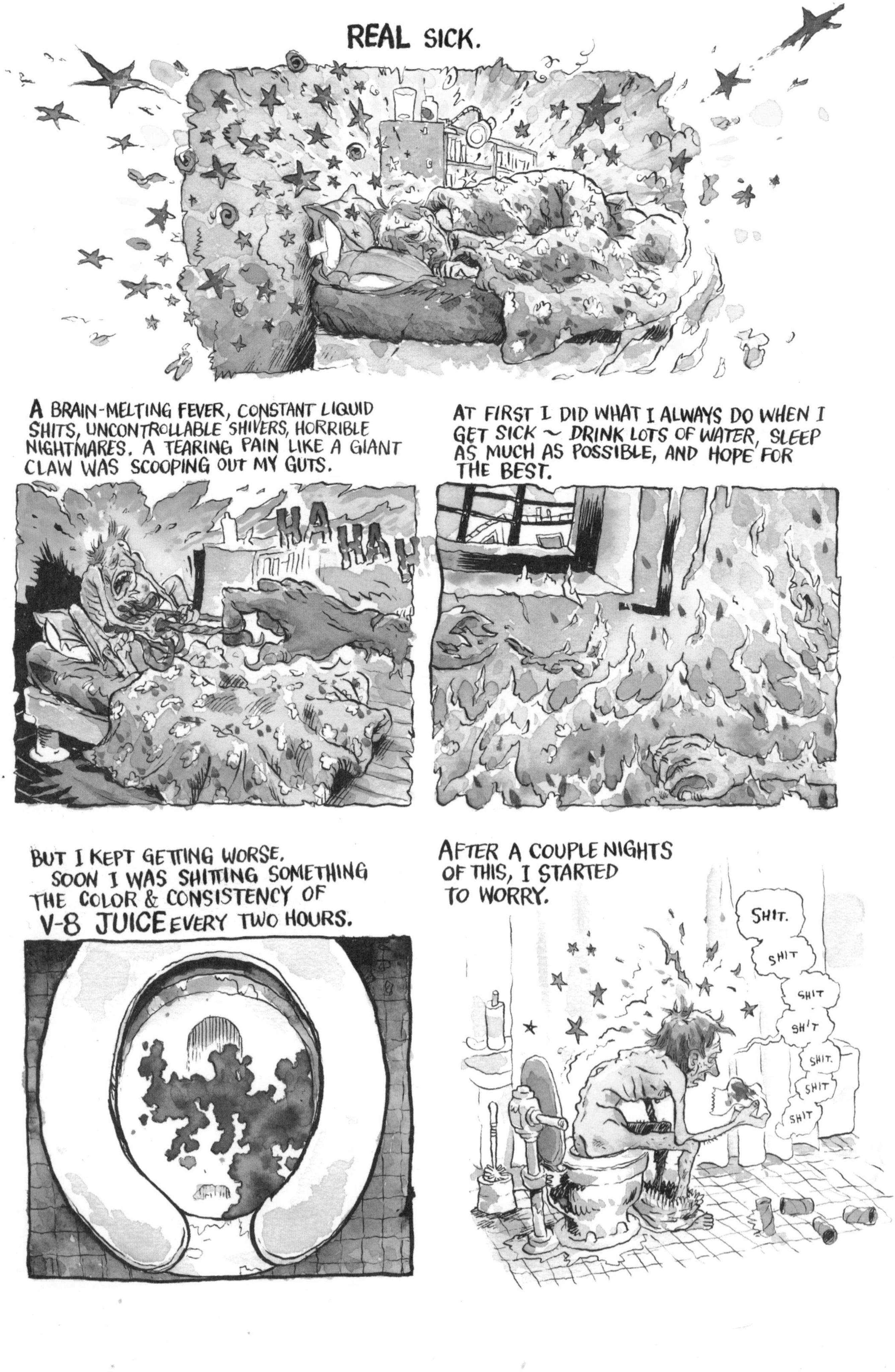
REAL SICK.
A BRAIN-MELTING FEVER, CONSTANT LIQUID SHITS, UNCONTROLLABLE SHIVERS, HORRIBLE NIGHTMARES. A TEARING PAIN LIKE A GIANT CLAW WAS SCOOPING OUT MY GUTS.
HA HA HAH
AT FIRST I DID WHAT I ALWAYS DO WHEN I GET SICK ~ DRINK LOTS OF WATER, SLEEP AS MUCH AS POSSIBLE, AND HOPE FOR THE BEST.
BUT I KEPT GETTING WORSE. SOON I WAS SHITTING SOMETHING THE COLOR & CONSISTENCY OF V-8 JUICE EVERY TWO HOURS.
AFTER A COUPLE NIGHTS OF THIS, I STARTED TO WORRY.
SHIT.
SHIT
SHIT
SHIT
SHIT.
SHIT
SHIT

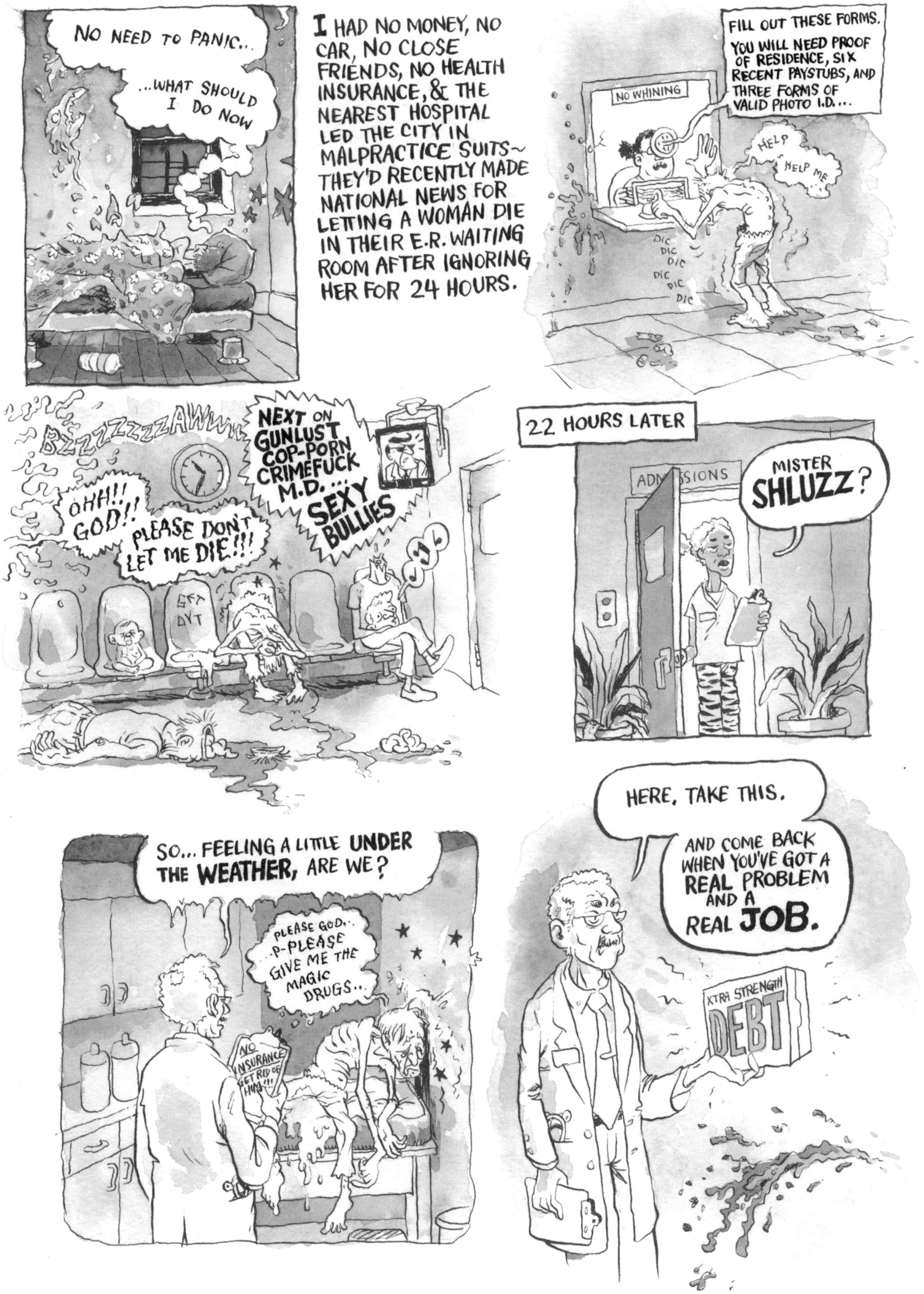

NO NEED TO PANIC...
...WHAT SHOULD I DO NOW
I HAD NO MONEY, NO CAR, NO CLOSE FRIENDS, NO HEALTH INSURANCE, & THE NEAREST HOSPITAL LED THE CITY IN MALPRACTICE SUITS~ THEY'D RECENTLY MADE NATIONAL NEWS FOR LETTING A WOMAN DIE IN THEIR E.R. WAITING ROOM AFTER IGNORING HER FOR 24 HOURS.
FILL OUT THESE FORMS.
YOU WILL NEED PROOF OF RESIDENCE, SIX RECENT PAYSTUBS, AND THREE FORMS OF VALID PHOTO I.D....
NO WHINING
HELP
HELP ME
DIC DIC DIC DIC DIC DIC
BZZZZZZZZAWWW
NEXT ON GUNLUST COP-PORN CRIMEFUCK M.D.... SEXY BULLIES
OHH!!! GOD!!
PLEASE DON'T LET ME DIE!!!
22 HOURS LATER
ADMISSIONS
MISTER SHLUZZ?
SO... FEELING A LITTLE UNDER THE WEATHER, ARE WE?
PLEASE GOD... P-PLEASE GIVE ME THE MAGIC DRUGS...
NO INSURANCE GET RID OF HIM!!!
HERE, TAKE THIS.
AND COME BACK WHEN YOU'VE GOT A REAL PROBLEM AND A REAL JOB.
XTRA STRENGTH DEBT

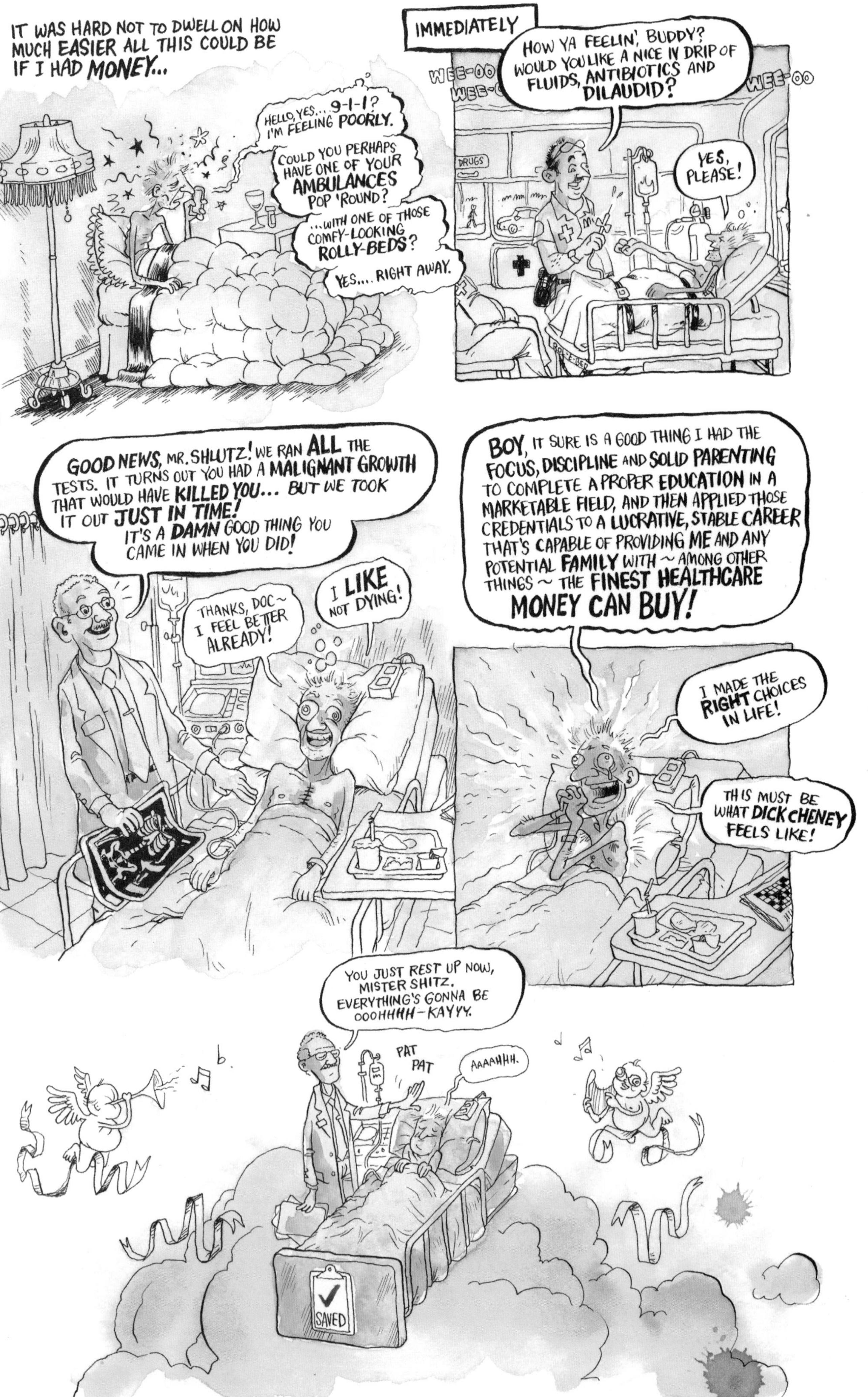

IT WAS HARD NOT TO DWELL ON HOW MUCH EASIER ALL THIS COULD BE IF I HAD MONEY...
HELLO, YES... 9-1-1? I'M FEELING POORLY.
COULD YOU PERHAPS HAVE ONE OF YOUR AMBULANCES POP 'ROUND?
...WITH ONE OF THOSE COMFY-LOOKING ROLLY-BEDS?
YES.... RIGHT AWAY.
IMMEDIATELY
WEE-OO WEE-OO
WEE-OO
HOW YA FEELIN', BUDDY? WOULD YOU LIKE A NICE IV DRIP OF FLUIDS, ANTIBIOTICS AND DILAUDID?
YES, PLEASE!
DRUGS
GOOD NEWS, MR. SHLUTZ! WE RAN ALL THE TESTS. IT TURNS OUT YOU HAD A MALIGNANT GROWTH THAT WOULD HAVE KILLED YOU... BUT WE TOOK IT OUT JUST IN TIME! IT'S A DAMN GOOD THING YOU CAME IN WHEN YOU DID!
THANKS, DOC~ I FEEL BETTER ALREADY!
I LIKE NOT DYING!
BOY, IT SURE IS A GOOD THING I HAD THE FOCUS, DISCIPLINE AND SOLID PARENTING TO COMPLETE A PROPER EDUCATION IN A MARKETABLE FIELD, AND THEN APPLIED THOSE CREDENTIALS TO A LUCRATIVE, STABLE CAREER THAT'S CAPABLE OF PROVIDING ME AND ANY POTENTIAL FAMILY WITH ~ AMONG OTHER THINGS ~ THE FINEST HEALTHCARE MONEY CAN BUY!
I MADE THE RIGHT CHOICES IN LIFE!
THIS MUST BE WHAT DICK CHENEY FEELS LIKE!
YOU JUST REST UP NOW, MISTER SHITZ. EVERYTHING'S GONNA BE OOOHHHH-KAYYY.
PAT PAT
AAAAHHH.
SAVED

DAYS & NIGHTS BLED TOGETHER IN MY BED, THE FEVER RISING AND THE DIARRHEA GETTING REDDER.

GRADUALLY MY WORRY & SELF-PITY DEGRADED DOWN TO A NULL, APATHETIC EXHAUSTION.*

OH GOD
OH GOD
OH GOD
OH GOD
OH GOD

I WAS DIMLY AWARE THAT THIS MAY BE GETTING SERIOUS ~ THAT MY BODY WOULDN'T BE GETTING BETTER ON ITS OWN.

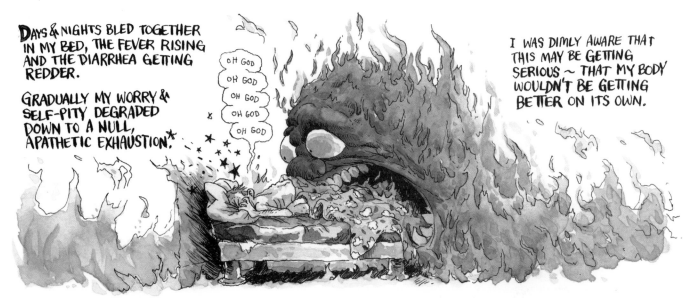

BUT **1.** I WAS TOO BROKE FOR AN UNINSURED HOSPITAL VISIT.

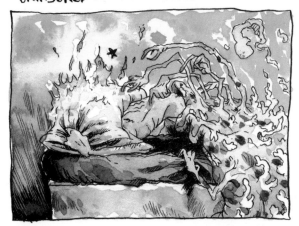

2. I REALIZED I WOULD RATHER DIE THAN MORTGAGE MY FUTURE TO AN ARM OF THE FOR-PROFIT HEALTHCARE INDUSTRY.

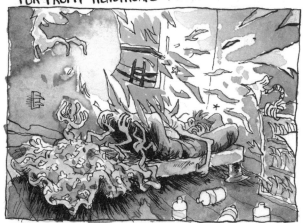

3. I'D ALSO RATHER DIE THAN INSULT MY FRIENDS OR ROOMMATES BY BEGGING THEM FOR HELP, SINCE I CAN'T BE BOTHERED TO RETURN THEIR PHONE CALLS & EMAILS WHEN I'M NOT ASKING THEM FOR FAVORS.

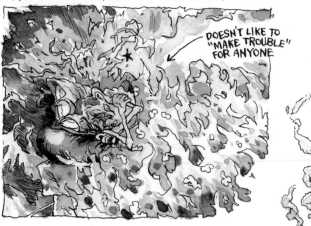

DOESN'T LIKE TO "MAKE TROUBLE" FOR ANYONE

4. I'M TOO VAIN & PETTY TO LET ANYONE SEE ME THIS HELPLESS ANYWAY. SO, WHAT DO I DO?

WHAT DO I DO?
WHAT DO I DO?
WHAT DO I DO?
WHAT DO I DO?

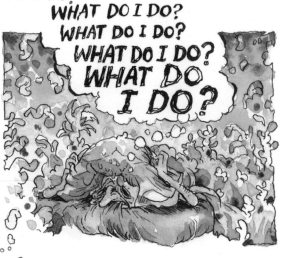

I LIE HERE IN THIS IKEA BED AND QUIETLY SHIT MYSELF TO DEATH.

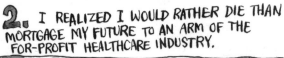

OUT OF COWARDICE, SHAME AND SELF-DISGUST.

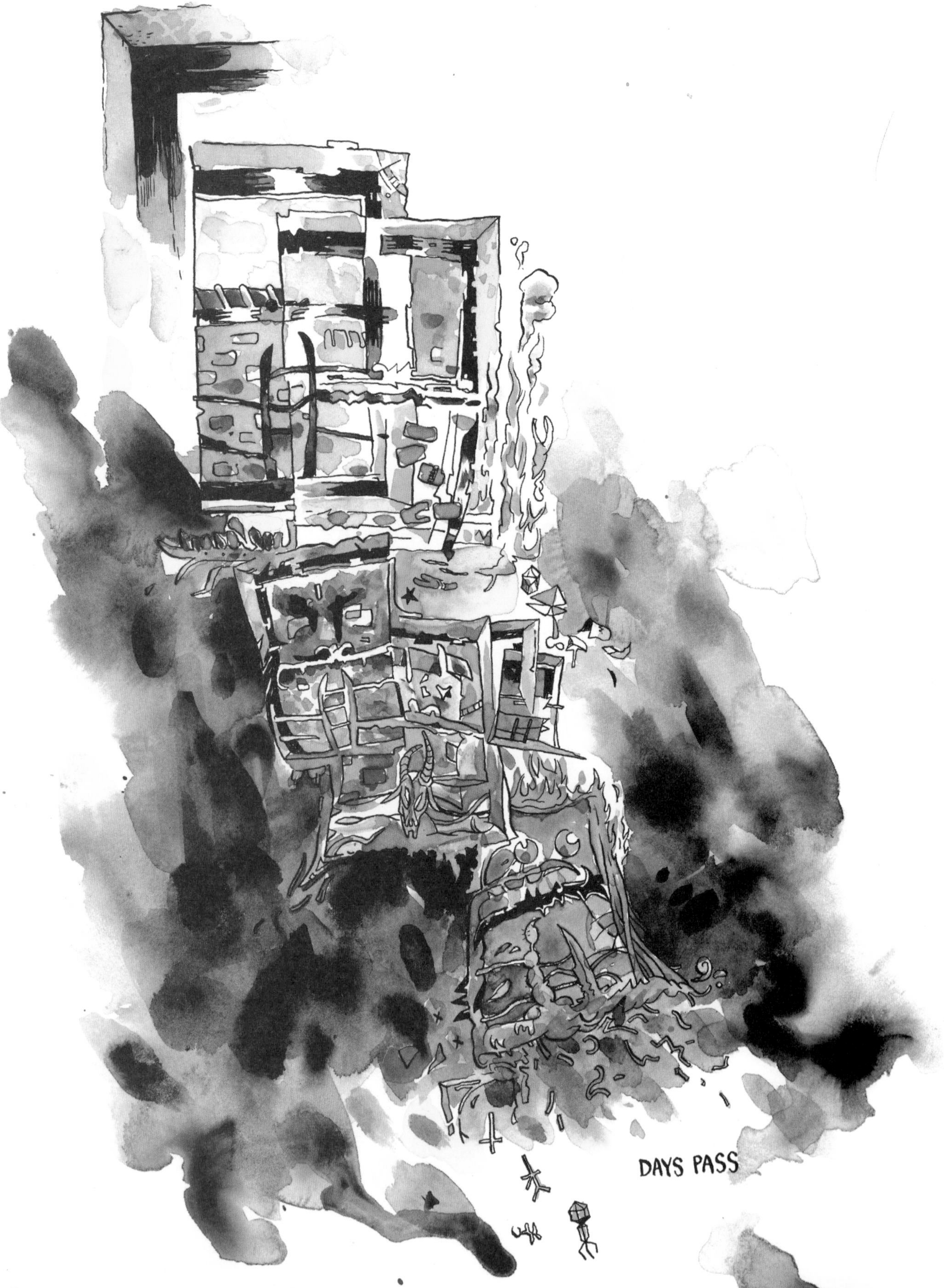
DAYS PASS

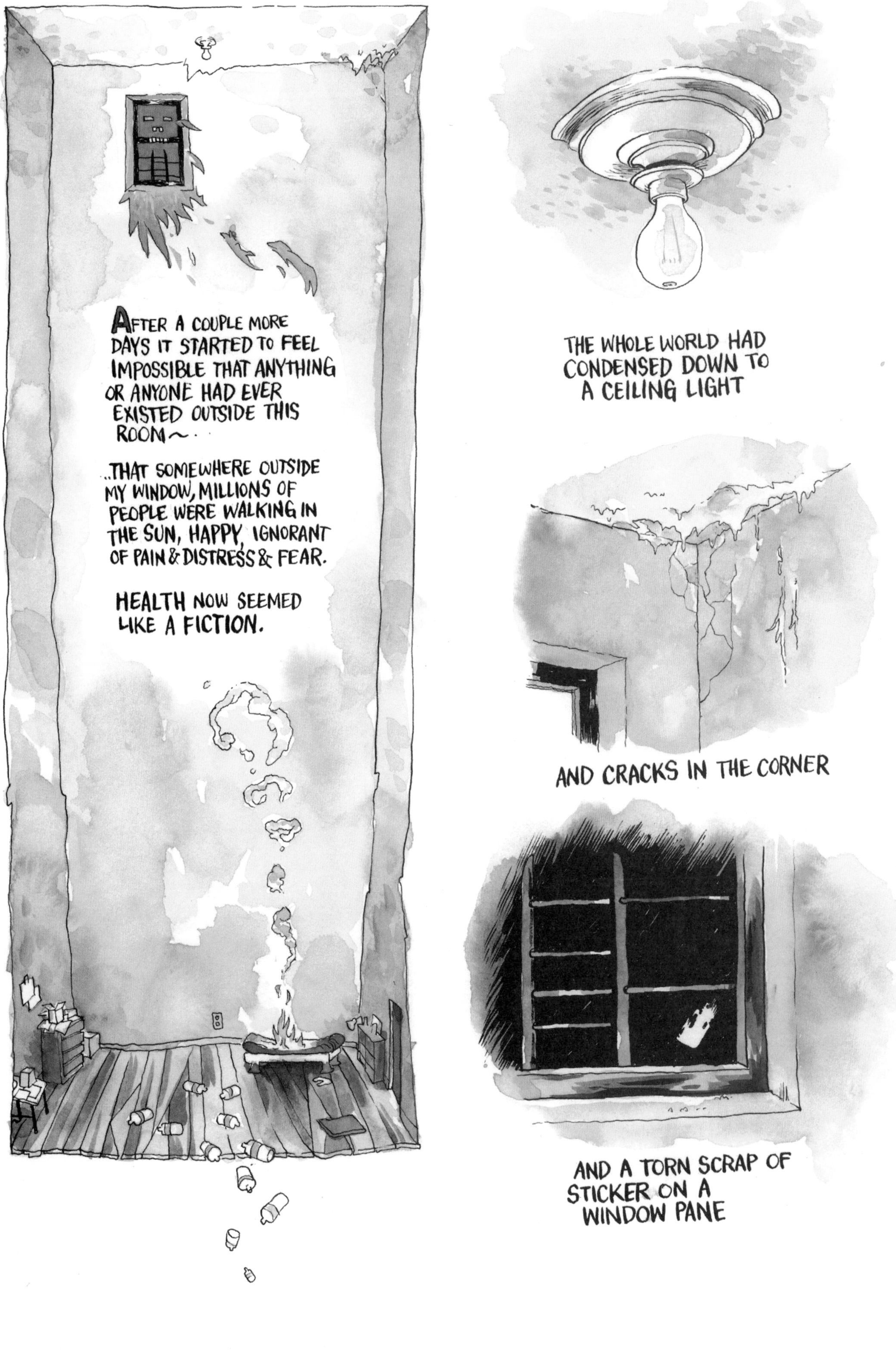
AFTER A COUPLE MORE DAYS IT STARTED TO FEEL IMPOSSIBLE THAT ANYTHING OR ANYONE HAD EVER EXISTED OUTSIDE THIS ROOM~.
..THAT SOMEWHERE OUTSIDE MY WINDOW, MILLIONS OF PEOPLE WERE WALKING IN THE SUN, HAPPY, IGNORANT OF PAIN & DISTRESS & FEAR.
HEALTH NOW SEEMED LIKE A FICTION.
THE WHOLE WORLD HAD CONDENSED DOWN TO A CEILING LIGHT
AND CRACKS IN THE CORNER
AND A TORN SCRAP OF STICKER ON A WINDOW PANE

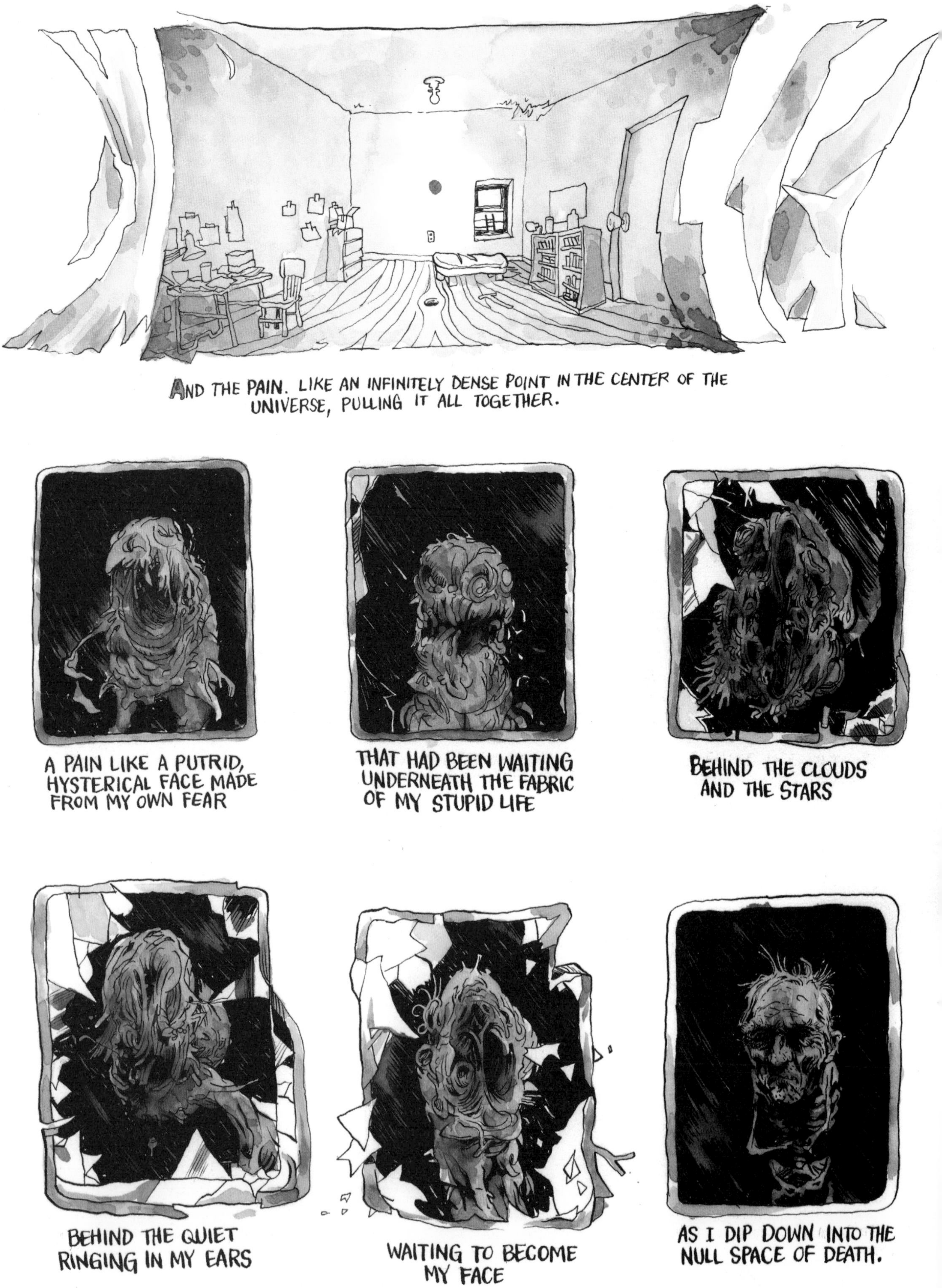
AND THE PAIN. LIKE AN INFINITELY DENSE POINT IN THE CENTER OF THE UNIVERSE, PULLING IT ALL TOGETHER.
A PAIN LIKE A PUTRID, HYSTERICAL FACE MADE FROM MY OWN FEAR
THAT HAD BEEN WAITING UNDERNEATH THE FABRIC OF MY STUPID LIFE
BEHIND THE CLOUDS AND THE STARS
BEHIND THE QUIET RINGING IN MY EARS
WAITING TO BECOME MY FACE
AS I DIP DOWN INTO THE NULL SPACE OF DEATH.

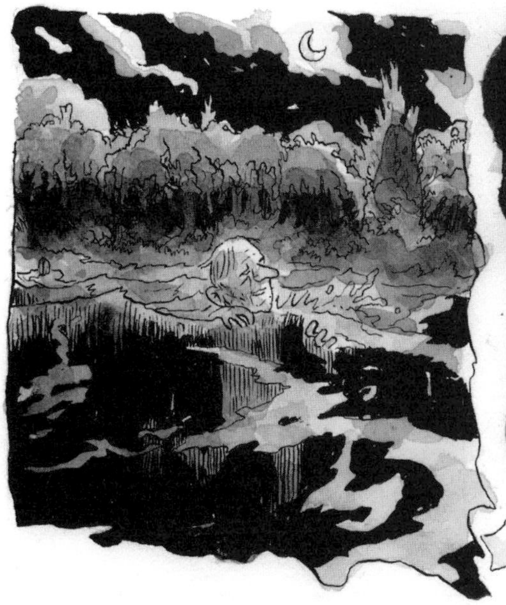

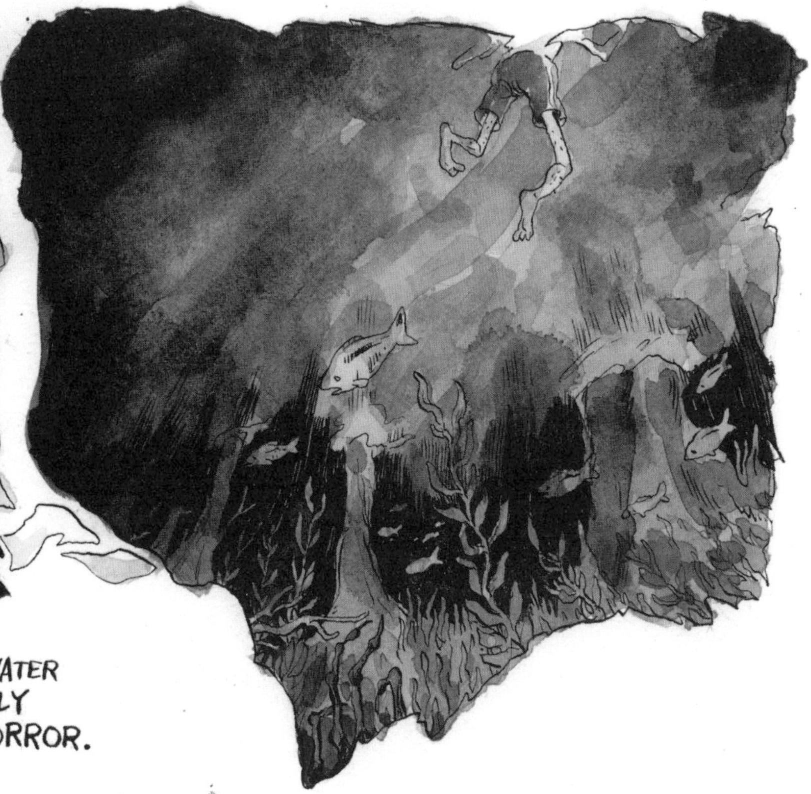

AFTER YEARS OF TREADING WATER
IN THE SHALLOWS, I'D FINALLY
BEEN SINGLED OUT BY HORROR.

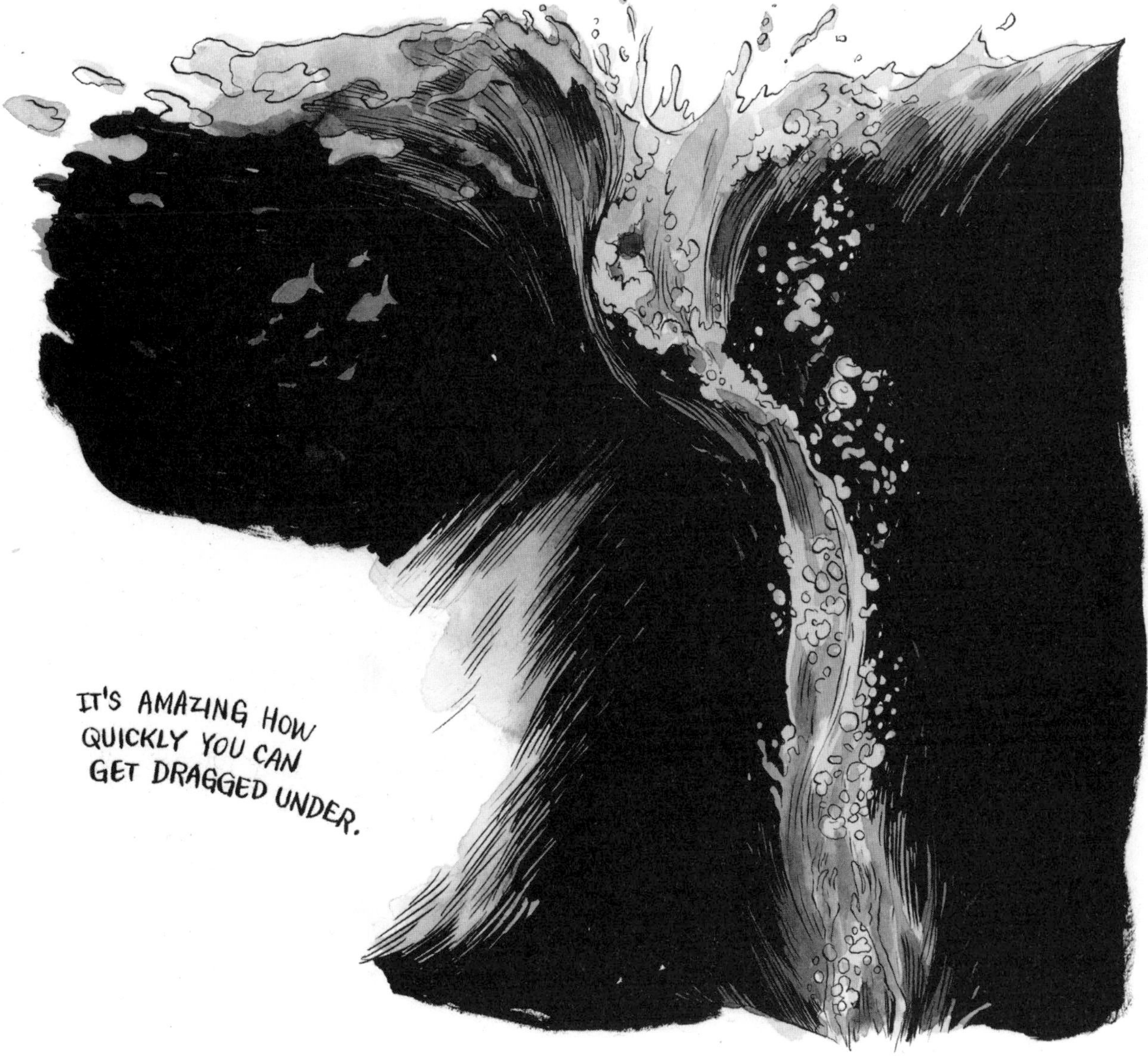
IT'S AMAZING HOW
QUICKLY YOU CAN
GET DRAGGED UNDER.

NO ONE ELSE I KNEW IN NEW YORK SEEMED TO HAVE ANY TROUBLE SURVIVING...

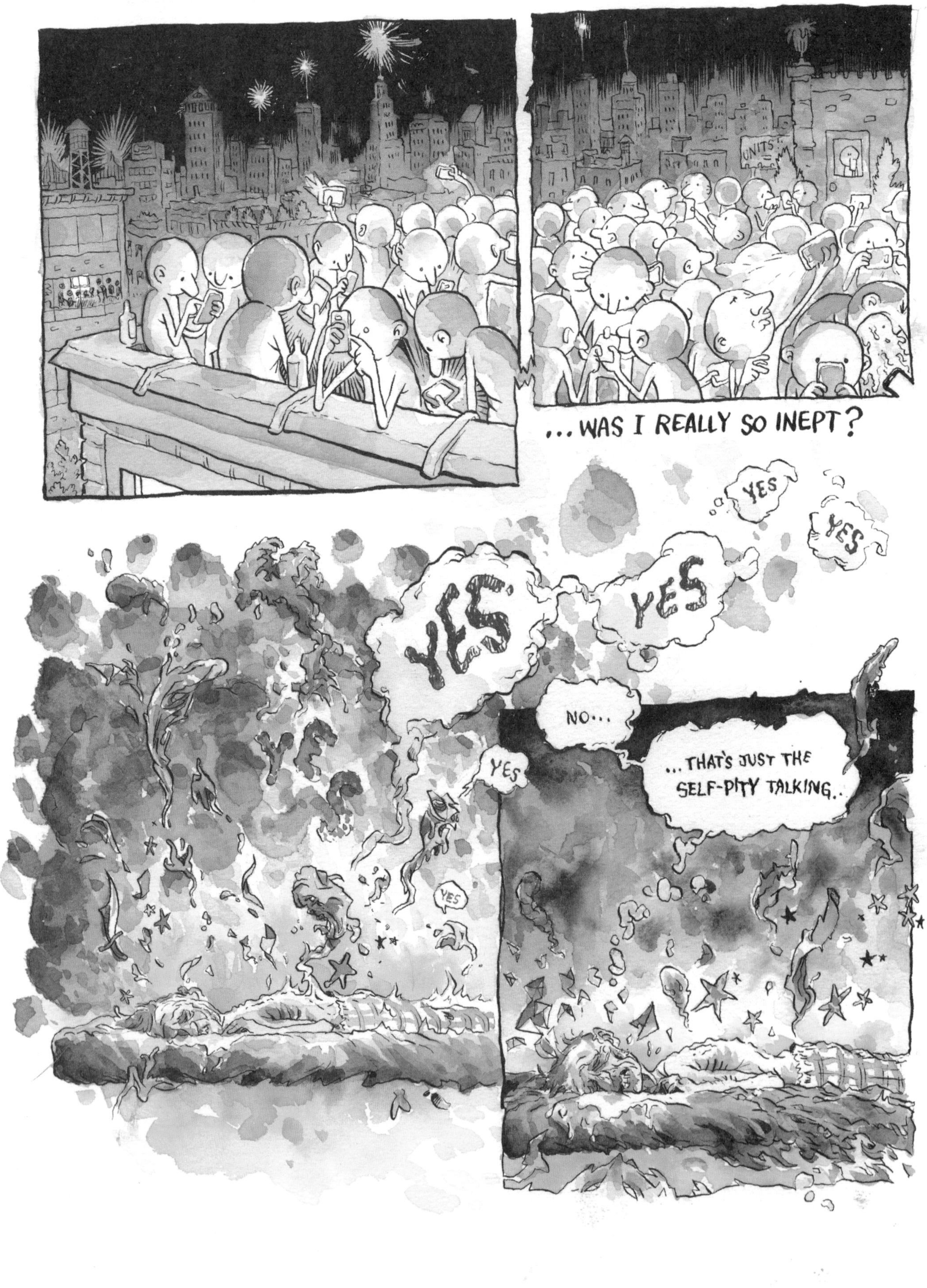
UNITS
...WAS I REALLY SO INEPT?
YES
YES
YES
YES
NO...
...THAT'S JUST THE SELF-PITY TALKING..
YES
YES

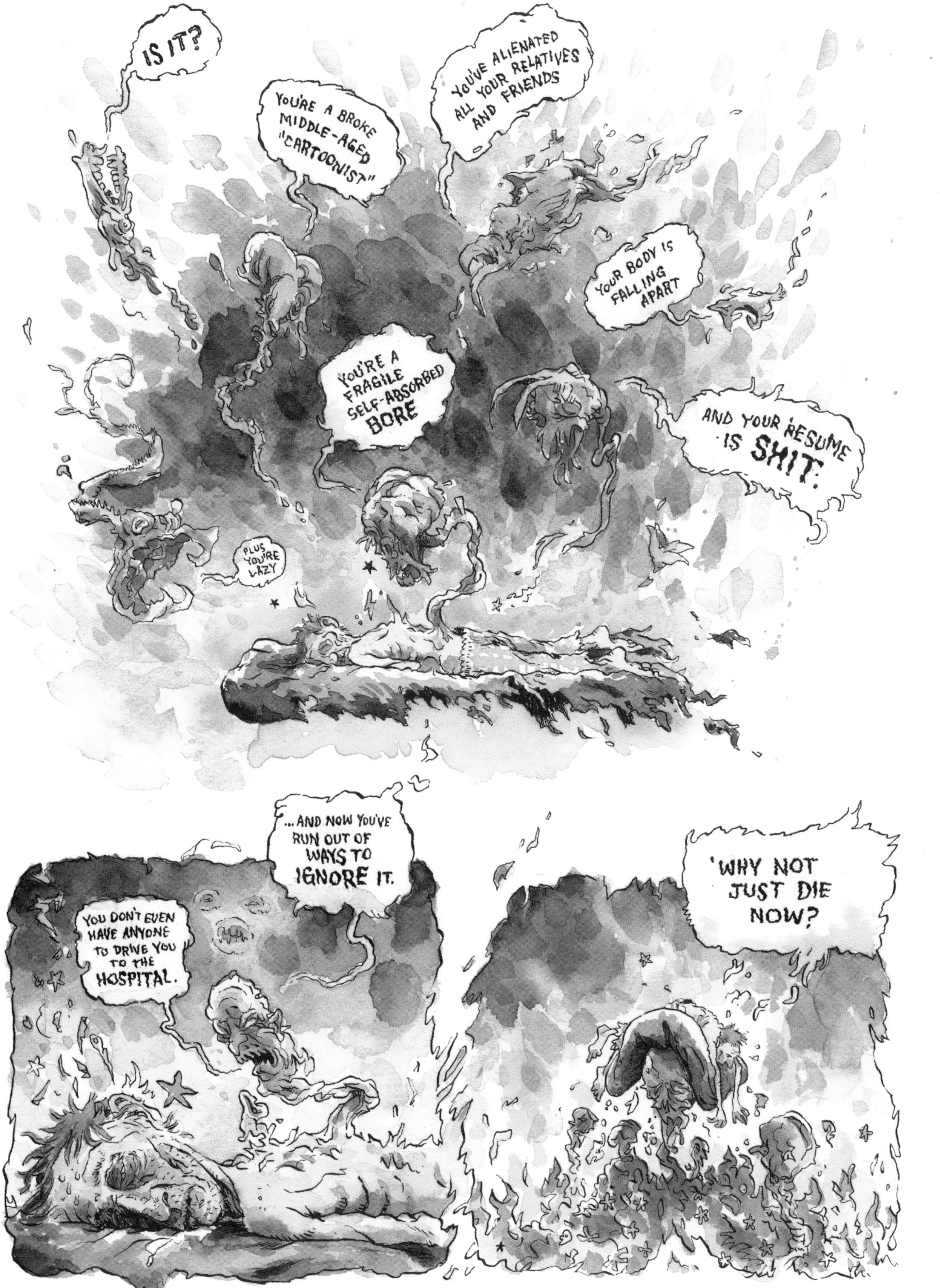
IS IT?
YOU'RE A BROKE MIDDLE-AGED "CARTOONIST"
YOU'VE ALIENATED ALL YOUR RELATIVES AND FRIENDS
YOUR BODY IS FALLING APART
YOU'RE A FRAGILE SELF-ABSORBED BORE
AND YOUR RESUME IS SHIT.
PLUS YOU'RE LAZY
YOU DON'T EVEN HAVE ANYONE TO DRIVE YOU TO THE HOSPITAL.
...AND NOW YOU'VE RUN OUT OF WAYS TO IGNORE IT.
'WHY NOT JUST DIE NOW?

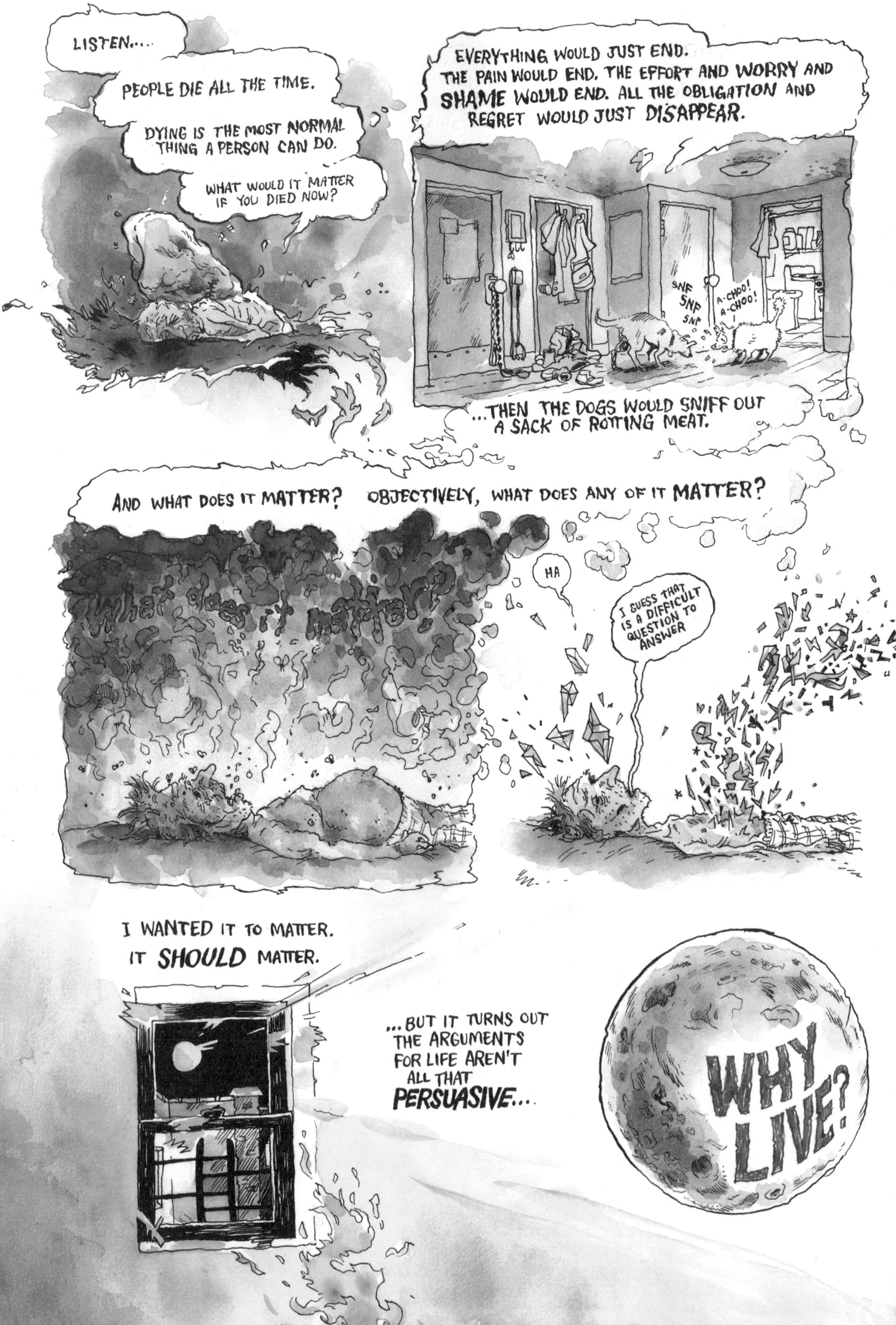
LISTEN....
PEOPLE DIE ALL THE TIME.
DYING IS THE MOST NORMAL THING A PERSON CAN DO.
WHAT WOULD IT MATTER IF YOU DIED NOW?
EVERYTHING WOULD JUST END. THE PAIN WOULD END. THE EFFORT AND WORRY AND SHAME WOULD END. ALL THE OBLIGATION AND REGRET WOULD JUST DISAPPEAR.
SNF SNF SNF
A-CHOO! A-CHOO!
...THEN THE DOGS WOULD SNIFF OUT A SACK OF ROTTING MEAT.
AND WHAT DOES IT MATTER? OBJECTIVELY, WHAT DOES ANY OF IT MATTER?
What does it matter?
HA
I GUESS THAT IS A DIFFICULT QUESTION TO ANSWER
I WANTED IT TO MATTER.
IT SHOULD MATTER.
...BUT IT TURNS OUT THE ARGUMENTS FOR LIFE AREN'T ALL THAT PERSUASIVE...
WHY LIVE?

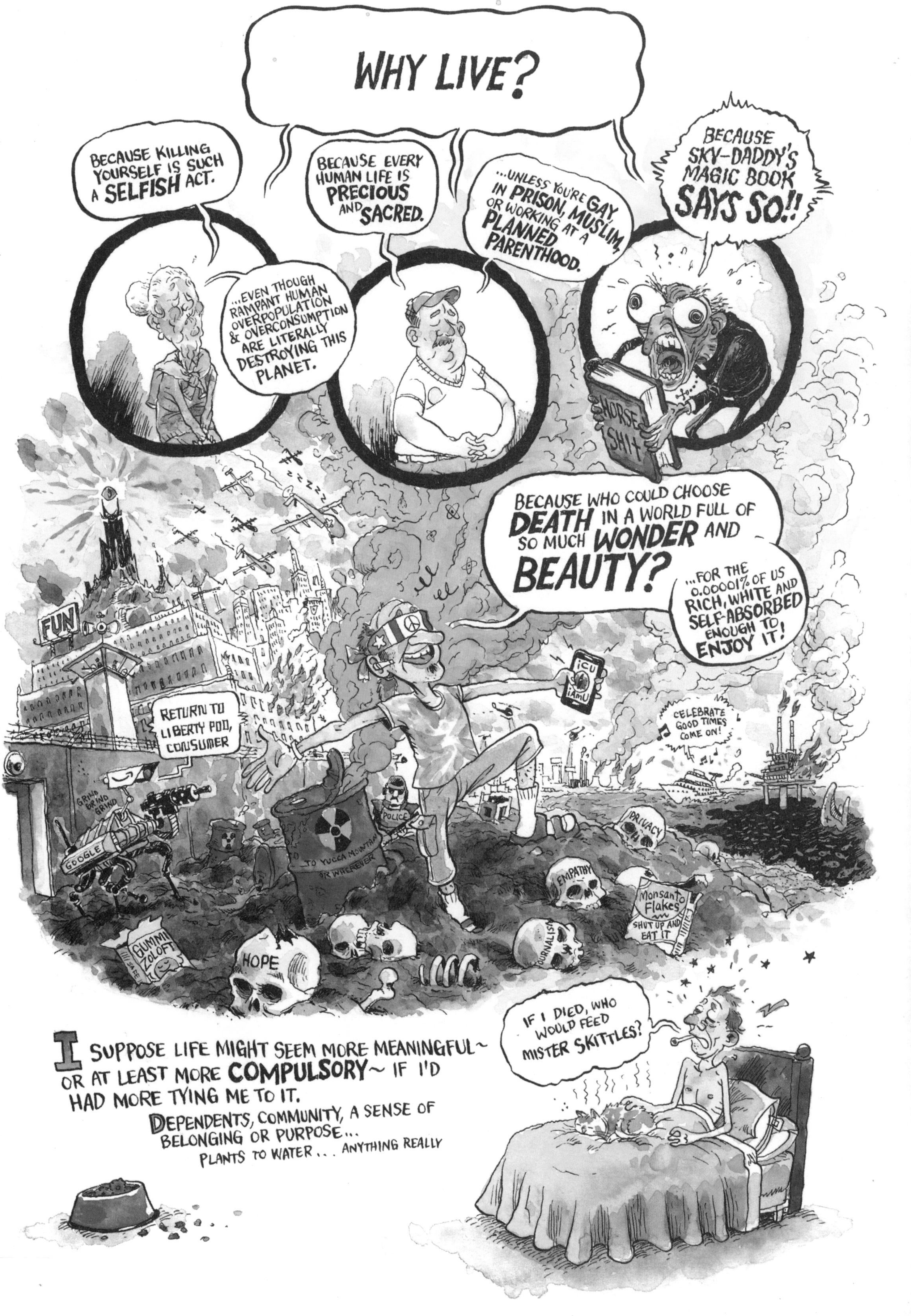
WHY LIVE?
BECAUSE KILLING YOURSELF IS SUCH A SELFISH ACT.
...EVEN THOUGH RAMPANT HUMAN OVERPOPULATION & OVERCONSUMPTION ARE LITERALLY DESTROYING THIS PLANET.
BECAUSE EVERY HUMAN LIFE IS PRECIOUS AND SACRED.
...UNLESS YOU'RE GAY, IN PRISON, MUSLIM, OR WORKING AT A PLANNED PARENTHOOD.
BECAUSE SKY-DADDY'S MAGIC BOOK SAYS SO!!
HORSE SHIT
BECAUSE WHO COULD CHOOSE DEATH IN A WORLD FULL OF SO MUCH WONDER AND BEAUTY?
...FOR THE 0.00001% OF US RICH, WHITE AND SELF-ABSORBED ENOUGH TO ENJOY IT!
FUN
RETURN TO LIBERTY POD, CONSUMER
ICU iAMU
CELEBRATE GOOD TIMES COME ON!
GRIND GRIND GRIND
GOOGLE
POLICE
TO YUCCA MOUNTAIN OR WHEREVER
PRIVACY
EMPATHY
Monsanto Flakes
SHUT UP AND EAT IT
JOURNALISM
HOPE
GUMMI ZOLOFT
IF I DIED, WHO WOULD FEED MISTER SKITTLES?
I SUPPOSE LIFE MIGHT SEEM MORE MEANINGFUL~ OR AT LEAST MORE COMPULSORY~ IF I'D HAD MORE TYING ME TO IT.
DEPENDENTS, COMMUNITY, A SENSE OF BELONGING OR PURPOSE...
PLANTS TO WATER... ANYTHING REALLY

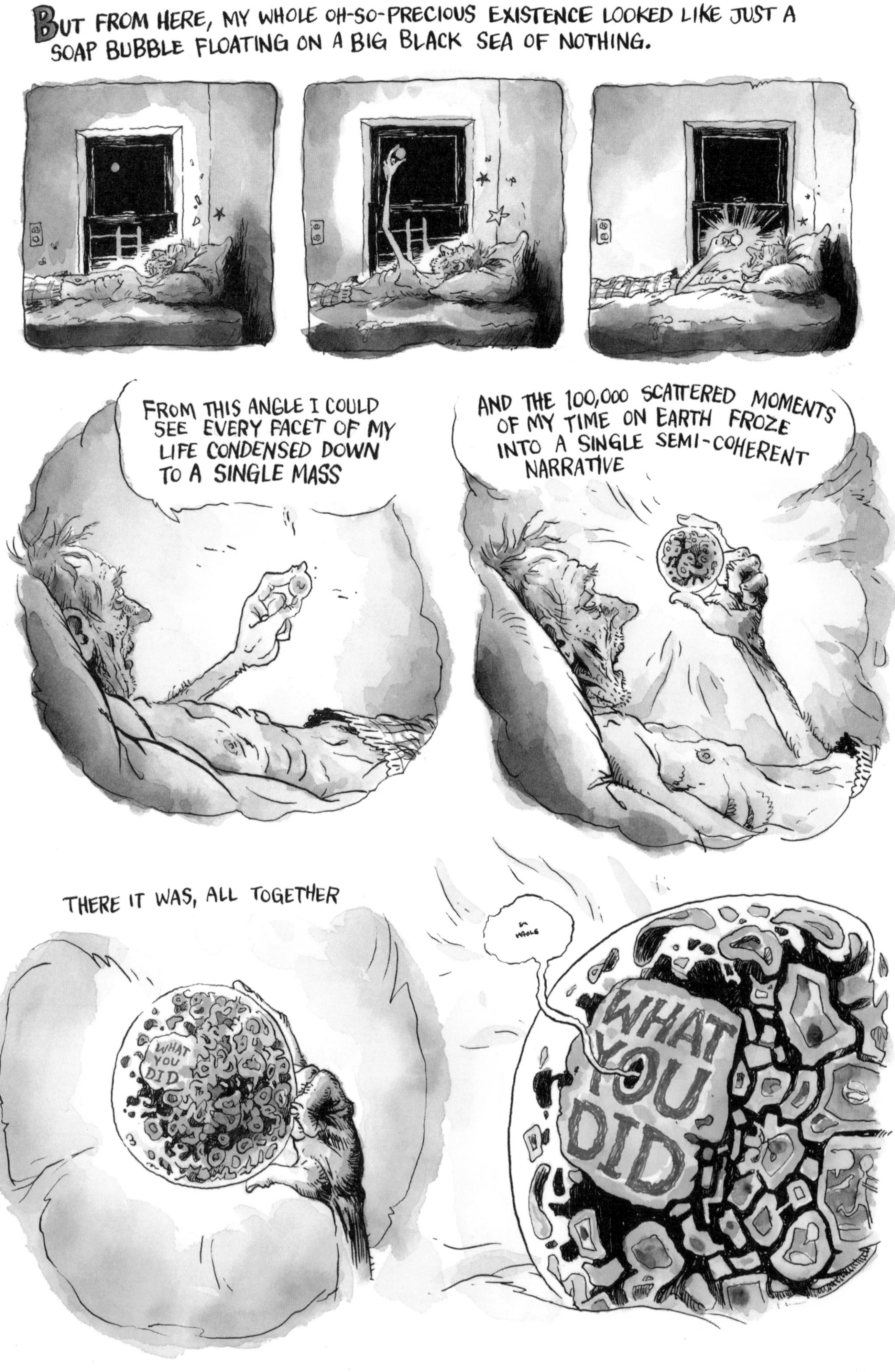
BUT FROM HERE, MY WHOLE OH-SO-PRECIOUS EXISTENCE LOOKED LIKE JUST A SOAP BUBBLE FLOATING ON A BIG BLACK SEA OF NOTHING.
FROM THIS ANGLE I COULD SEE EVERY FACET OF MY LIFE CONDENSED DOWN TO A SINGLE MASS
AND THE 100,000 SCATTERED MOMENTS OF MY TIME ON EARTH FROZE INTO A SINGLE SEMI-COHERENT NARRATIVE
THERE IT WAS, ALL TOGETHER
WHAT YOU DID
WHAT YOU DID

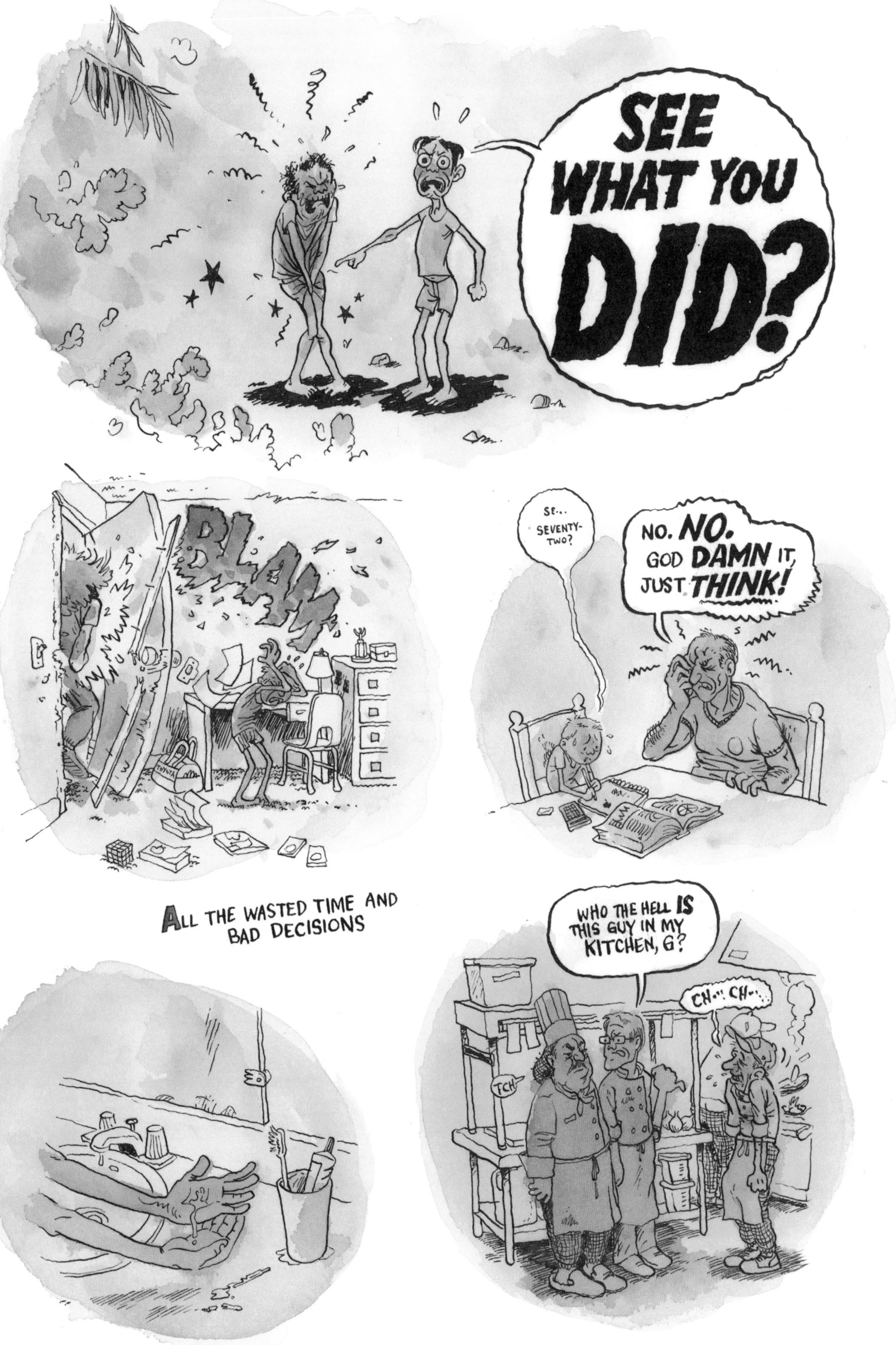
SEE WHAT YOU DID?
BLAM
SE... SEVENTY-TWO?
NO. NO. GOD DAMN IT, JUST THINK!
ALL THE WASTED TIME AND BAD DECISIONS
WHO THE HELL IS THIS GUY IN MY KITCHEN, G?
TCH
CH... CH...

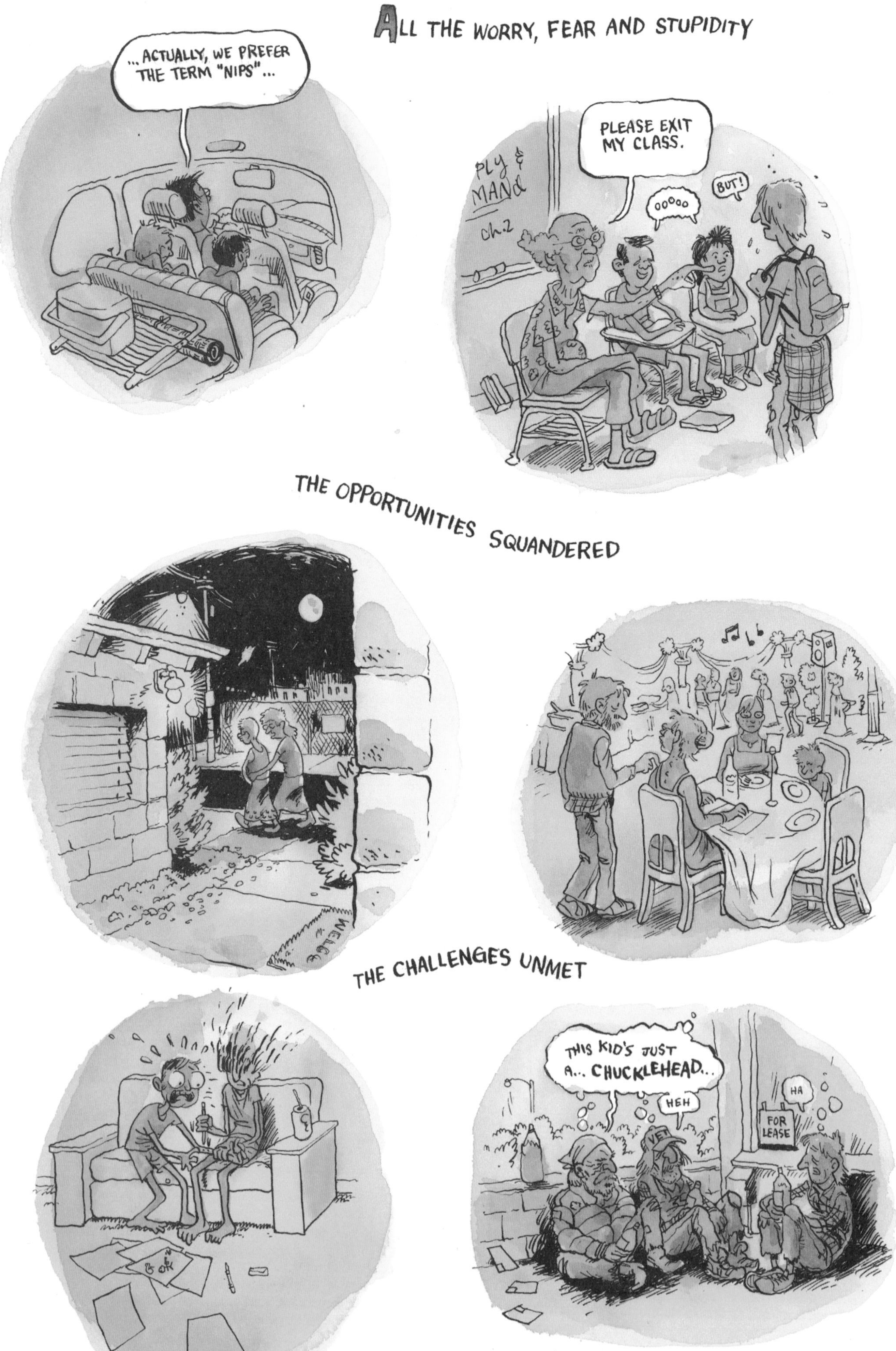
ALL THE WORRY, FEAR AND STUPIDITY
...ACTUALLY, WE PREFER THE TERM "NIPS"...
PLY & MAND
ch.2
PLEASE EXIT MY CLASS.
OOOOO
BUT!
THE OPPORTUNITIES SQUANDERED
THE CHALLENGES UNMET
THIS KID'S JUST A... CHUCKLEHEAD...
HEH
HA
FOR LEASE

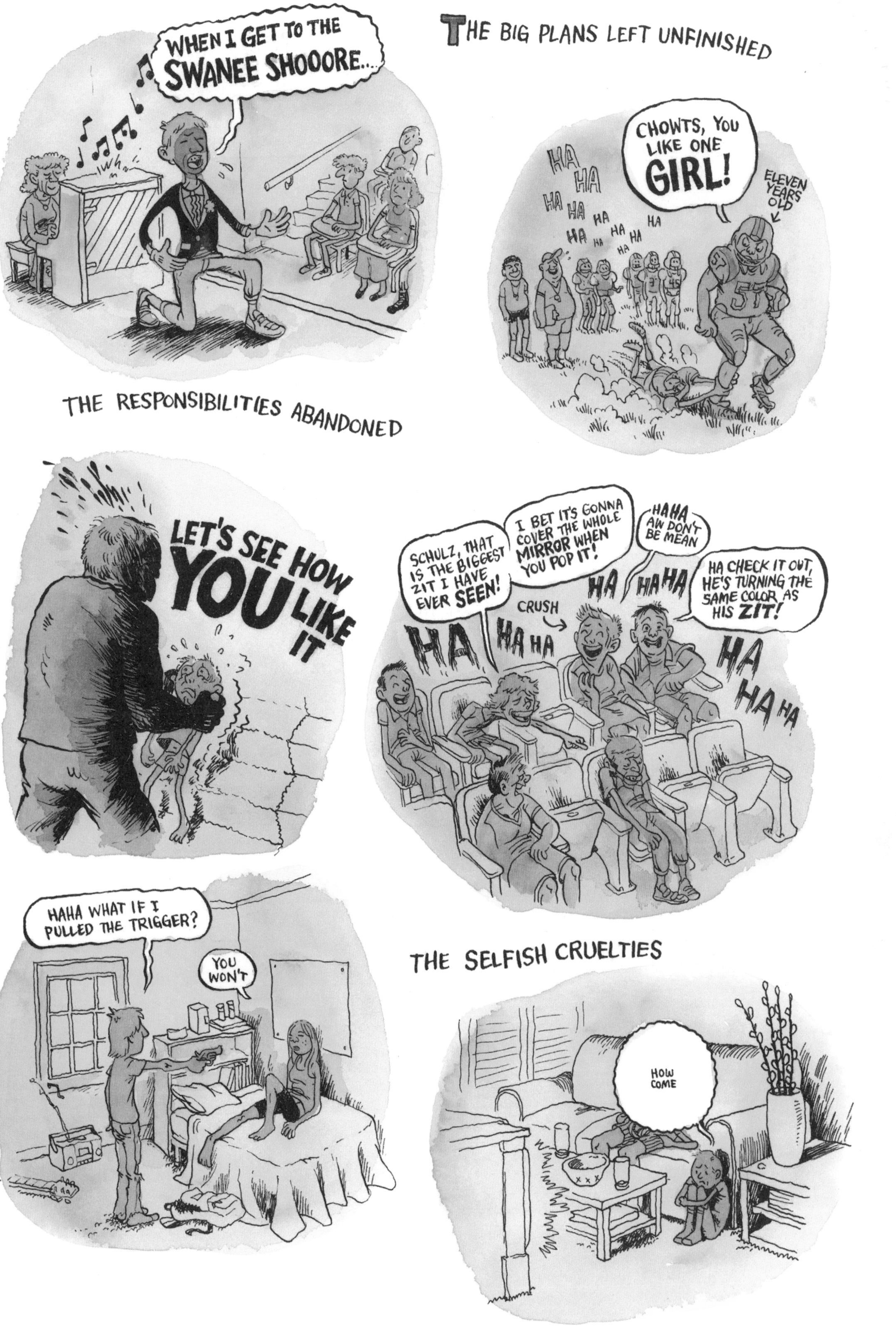
WHEN I GET TO THE SWANEE SHOOORE...
THE BIG PLANS LEFT UNFINISHED
CHOWTS, YOU LIKE ONE GIRL!
ELEVEN YEARS OLD
HA HA HA HA HA HA HA HA HA HA HA HA
THE RESPONSIBILITIES ABANDONED
LET'S SEE HOW YOU LIKE IT
SCHULZ, THAT IS THE BIGGEST ZIT I HAVE EVER SEEN!
I BET IT'S GONNA COVER THE WHOLE MIRROR WHEN YOU POP IT!
HAHA AW DON'T BE MEAN
HA CHECK IT OUT, HE'S TURNING THE SAME COLOR AS HIS ZIT!
CRUSH
HA HA HA HA HAHA HA HA HA
HAHA WHAT IF I PULLED THE TRIGGER?
YOU WON'T
THE SELFISH CRUELTIES
HOW COME

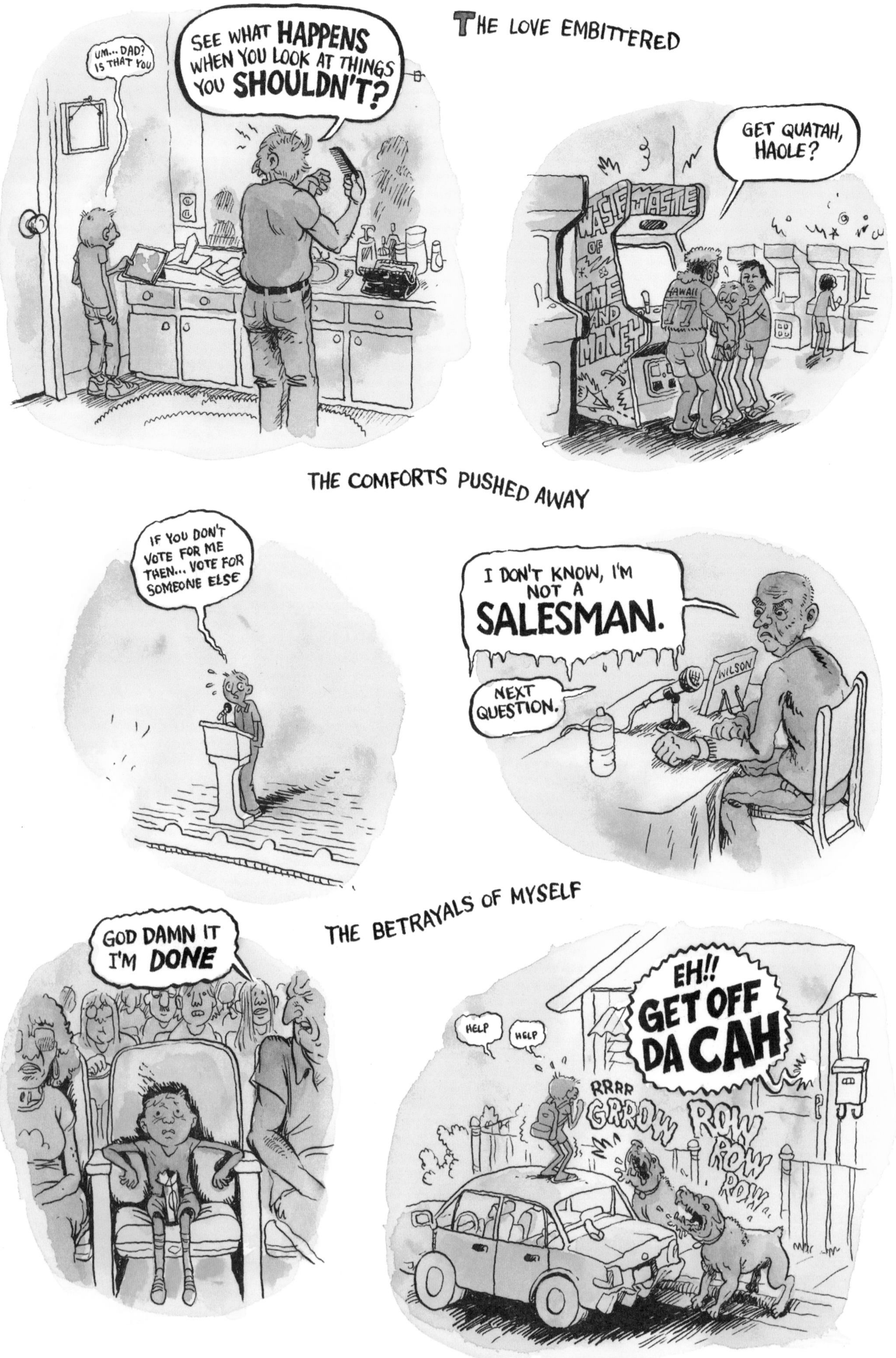
THE LOVE EMBITTERED
UM... DAD? IS THAT YOU
SEE WHAT HAPPENS WHEN YOU LOOK AT THINGS YOU SHOULDN'T?
WASTE OF TIME AND MONEY
HAWAII 77
GET QUATAH, HAOLE?
THE COMFORTS PUSHED AWAY
IF YOU DON'T VOTE FOR ME THEN... VOTE FOR SOMEONE ELSE
I DON'T KNOW, I'M NOT A SALESMAN.
NEXT QUESTION.
WILSON
THE BETRAYALS OF MYSELF
GOD DAMN IT I'M DONE
HELP
HELP
EH!! GET OFF DA CAH
RRRR
GRROW
ROW
ROW
ROW

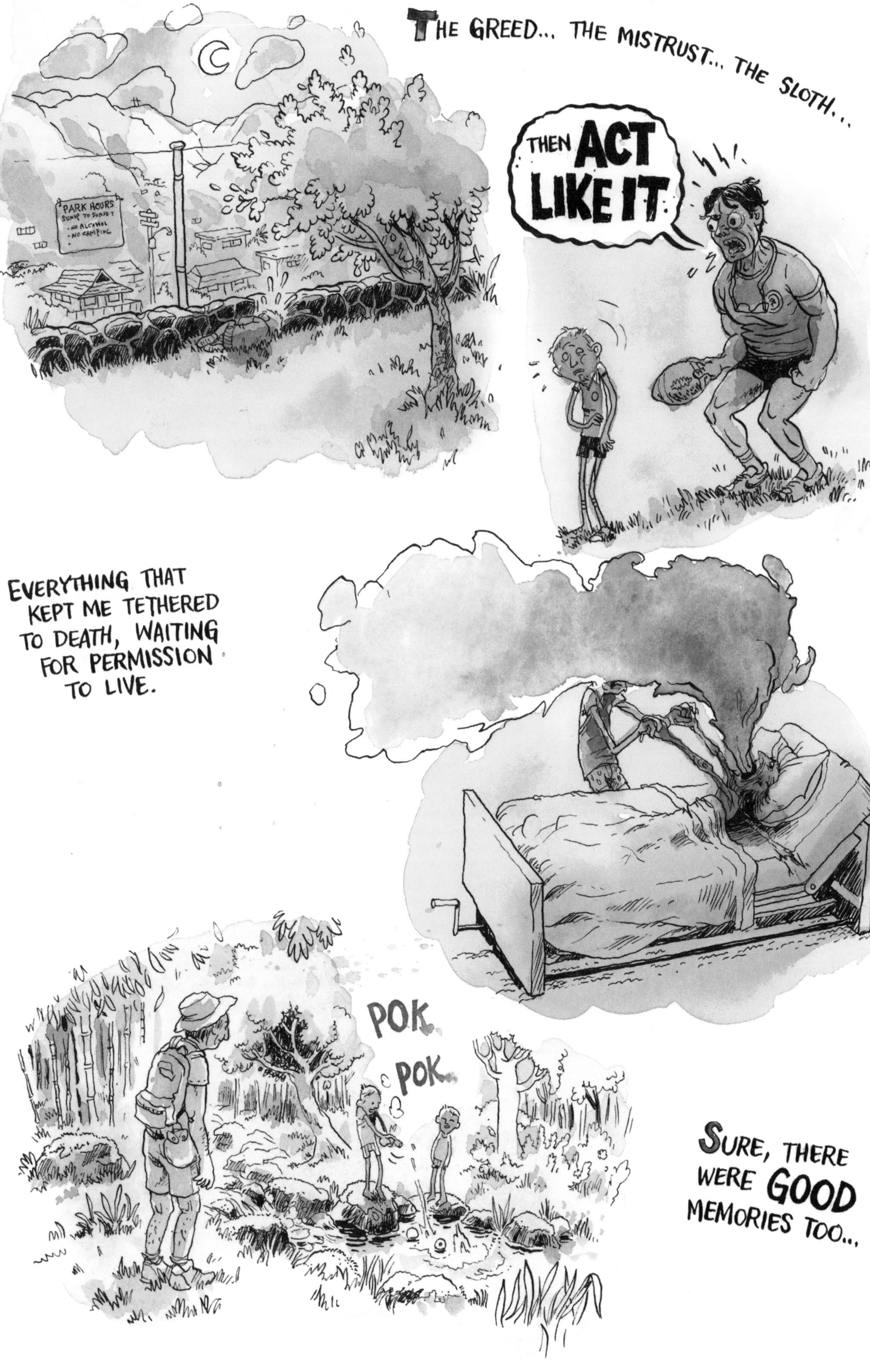
THE GREED... THE MISTRUST... THE SLOTH...
PARK HOURS
SUNUP TO SUNSET
• NO ALCOHOL
• NO CAMPING
THEN ACT LIKE IT
EVERYTHING THAT KEPT ME TETHERED TO DEATH, WAITING FOR PERMISSION TO LIVE.
POK
POK
SURE, THERE WERE GOOD MEMORIES TOO...

VALIDATION... JOY... COMMUNION...

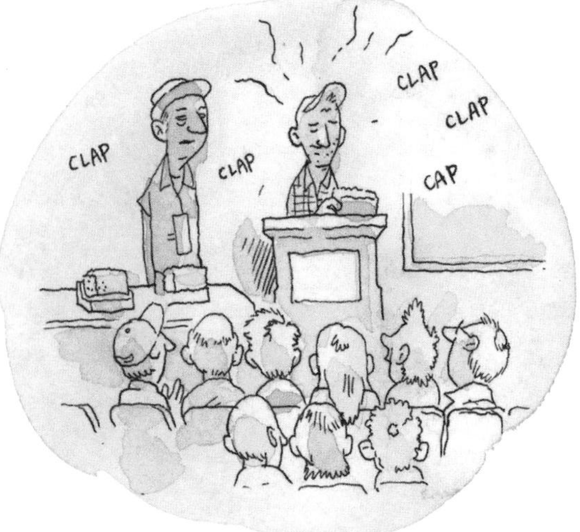
CLAP
CLAP
CLAP
CLAP
CAP

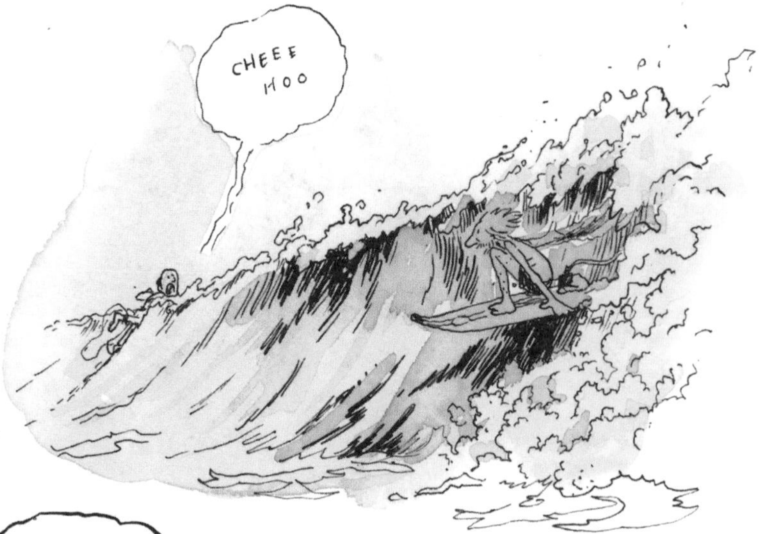
CHEEE HOO

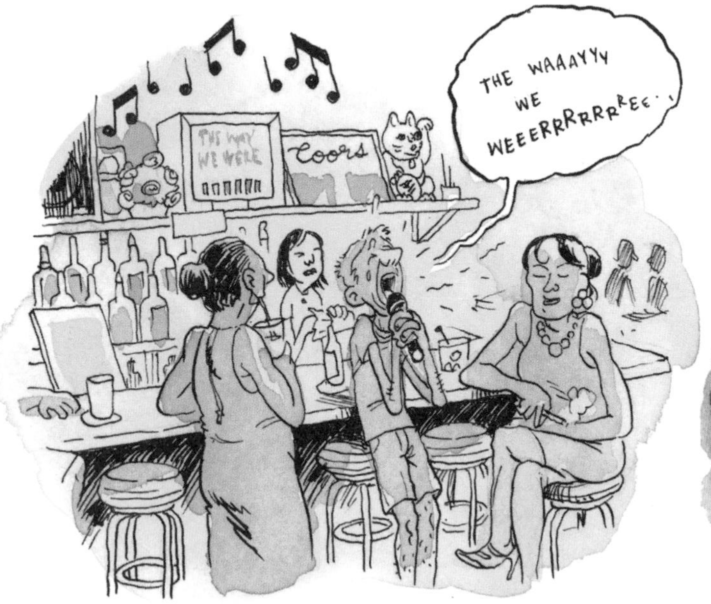
THE WAAAYYY WE WEEERRRRRREE...
Coors

BUT THESE DIDN'T HOVER OVER MY BED EVERY NIGHT

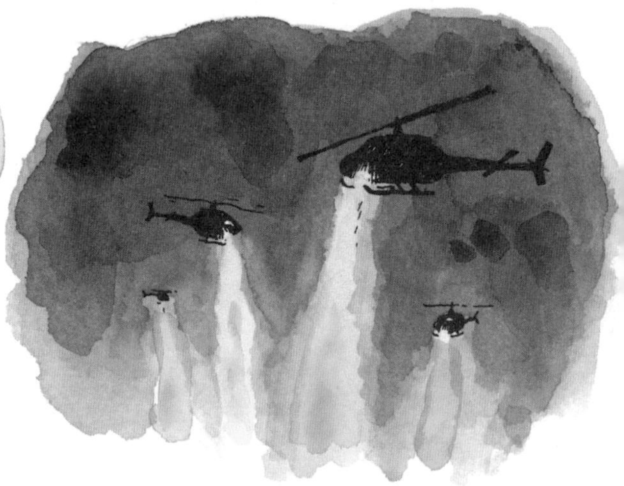

DEMANDING AN EXPLANATION

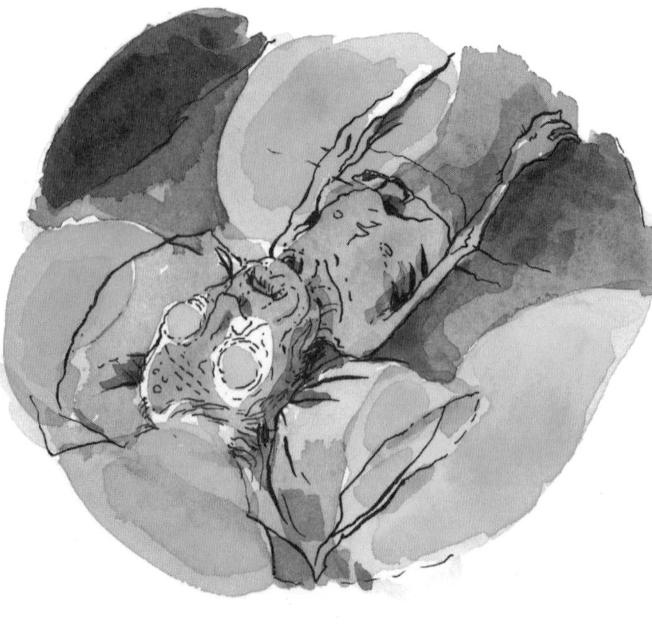

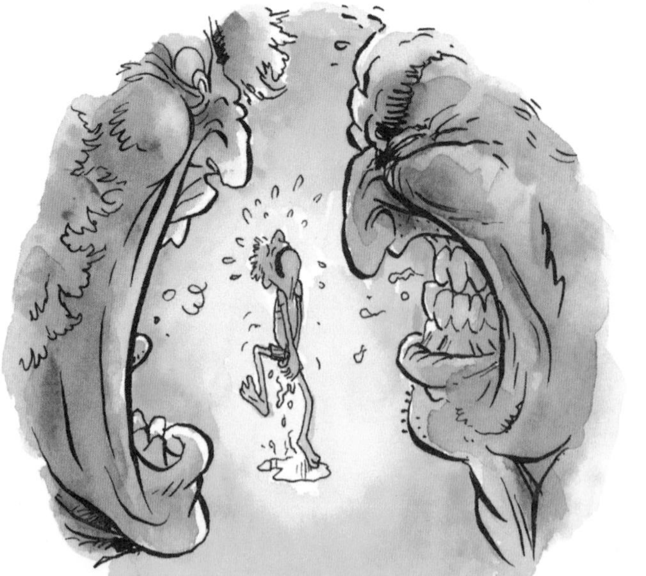

THERE WAS JUST SO MUCH **MORE** OF THE BAD.

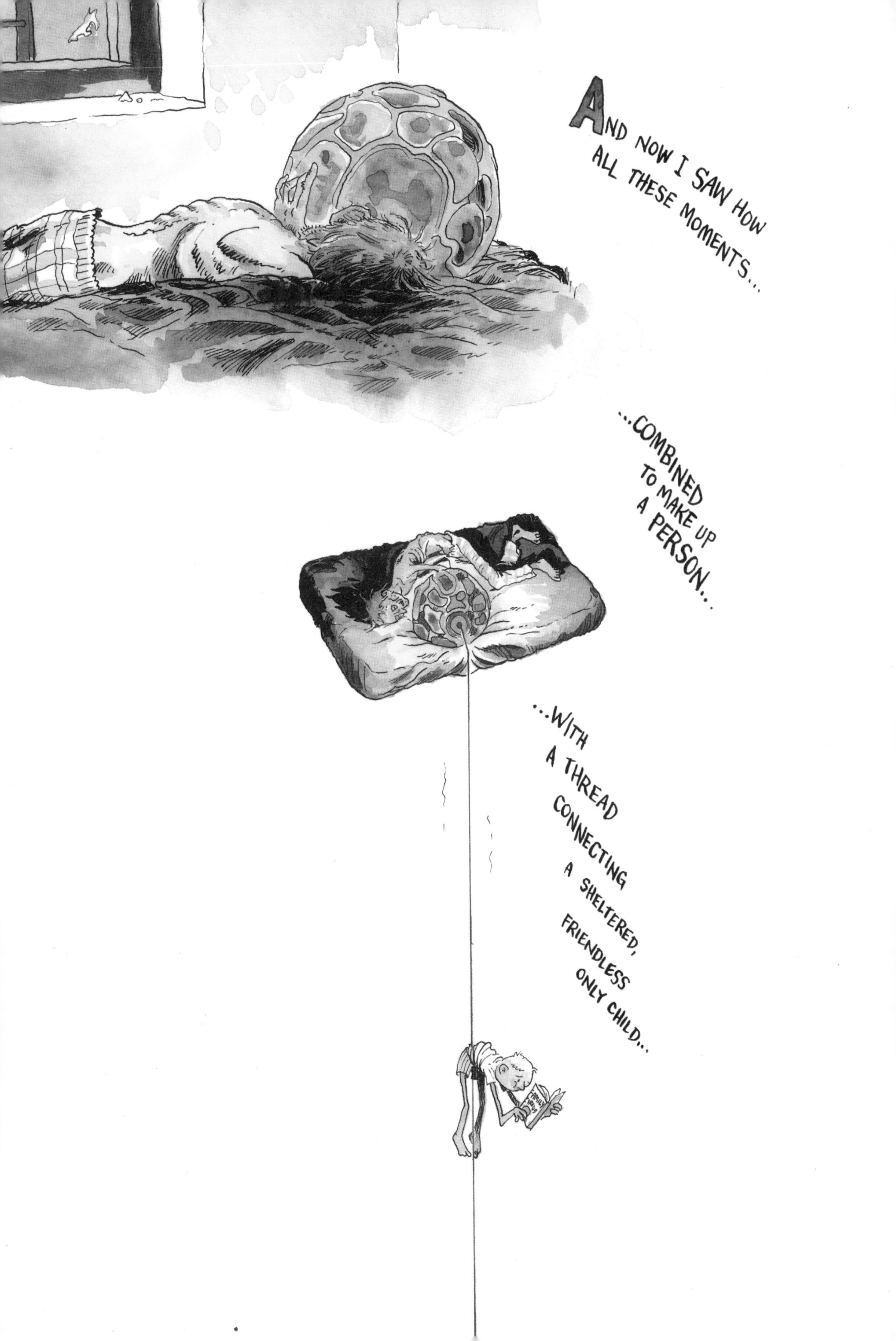
AND NOW I SAW HOW ALL THESE MOMENTS...
...COMBINED TO MAKE UP A PERSON...
...WITH A THREAD CONNECTING A SHELTERED, FRIENDLESS ONLY CHILD...

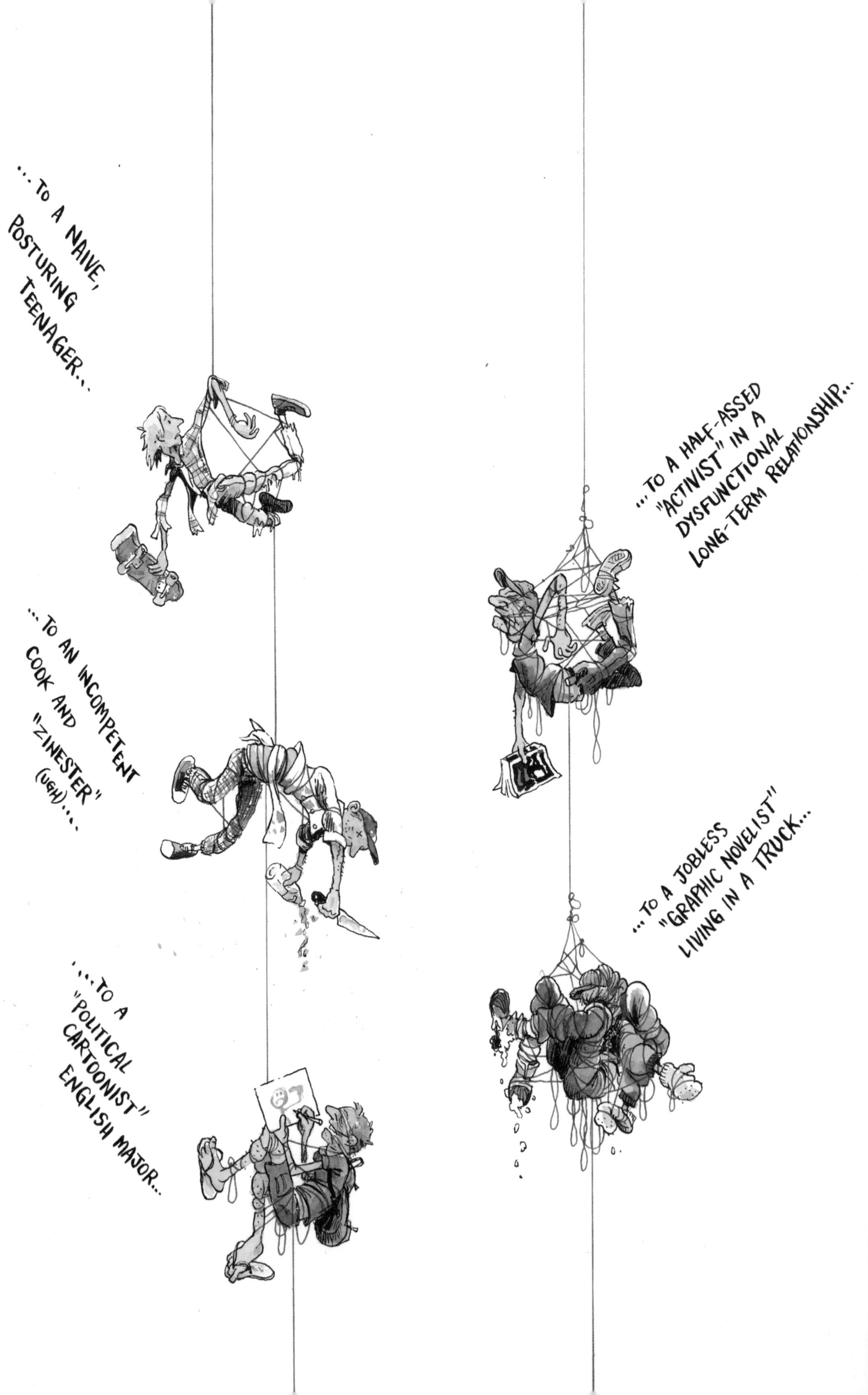
...TO A NAIVE, POSTURING TEENAGER...
...TO AN INCOMPETENT COOK AND "ZINESTER" (UGH)...
..."TO A "POLITICAL CARTOONIST" ENGLISH MAJOR...
...TO A HALF-ASSED "ACTIVIST" IN A DYSFUNCTIONAL LONG-TERM RELATIONSHIP...
...TO A JOBLESS "GRAPHIC NOVELIST" LIVING IN A TRUCK...

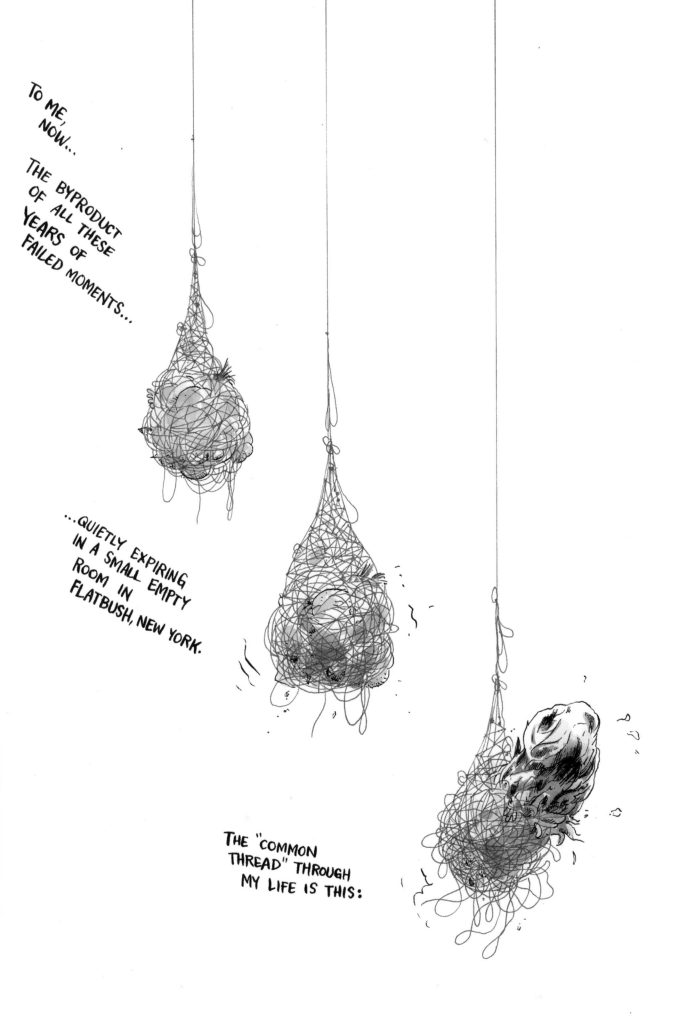

TO ME,
NOW...

THE BYPRODUCT
OF ALL THESE
YEARS OF
FAILED MOMENTS...

...QUIETLY EXPIRING
IN A SMALL EMPTY
ROOM IN
FLATBUSH, NEW YORK.

THE "COMMON
THREAD" THROUGH
MY LIFE IS THIS:

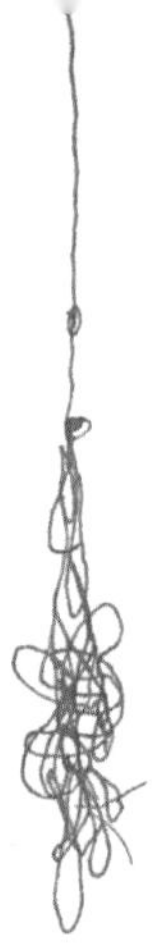

"I" DON'T EXIST.

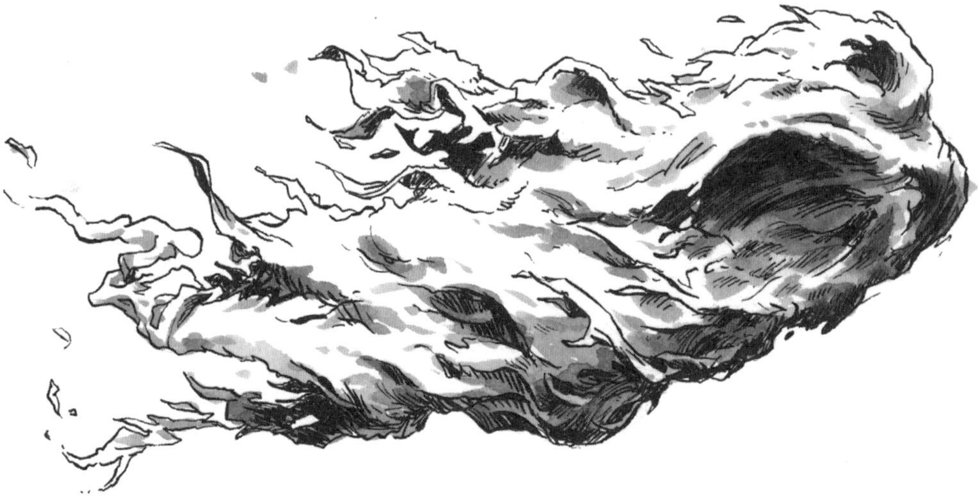

I'M A GHOST. A PSYCHIC STILLBIRTH.

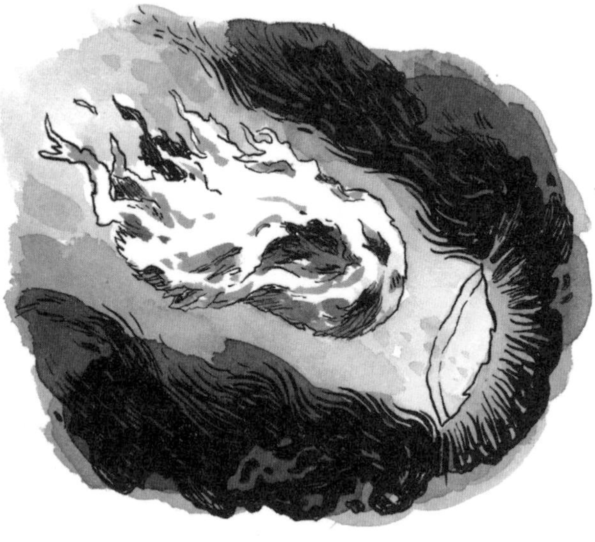

HAUNTING FOUR DECADES OF EMPTY ROOMS

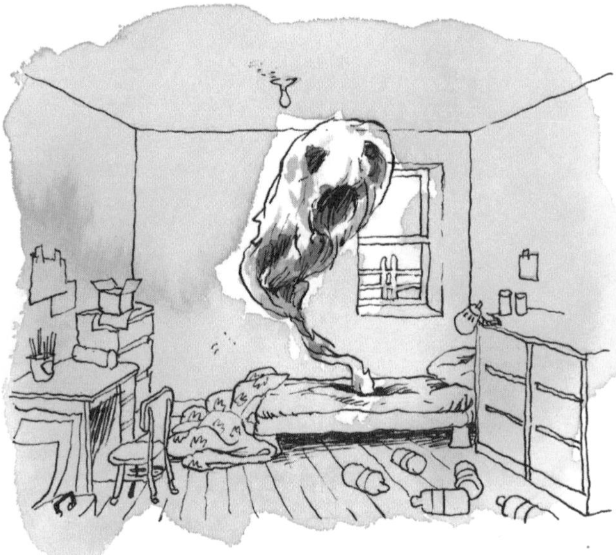

WAITING DUMBLY FOR ITS LIFE TO BEGIN.

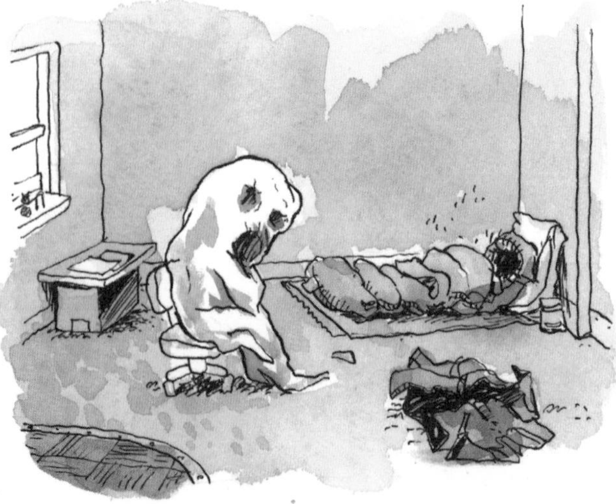

NO PLANS MADE, NO BONDS FORMED.

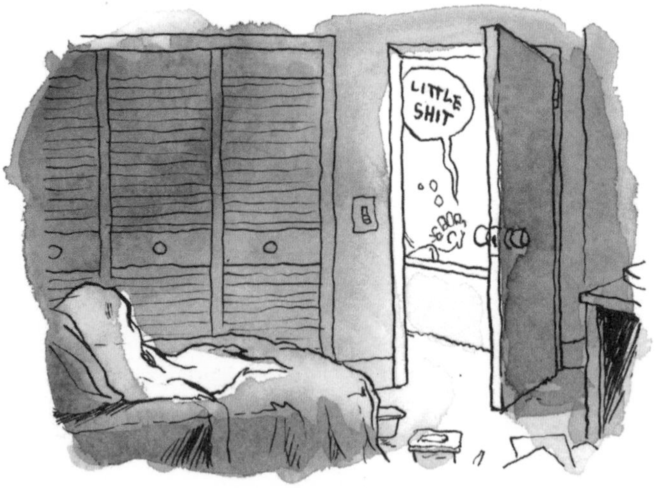
LITTLE SHIT

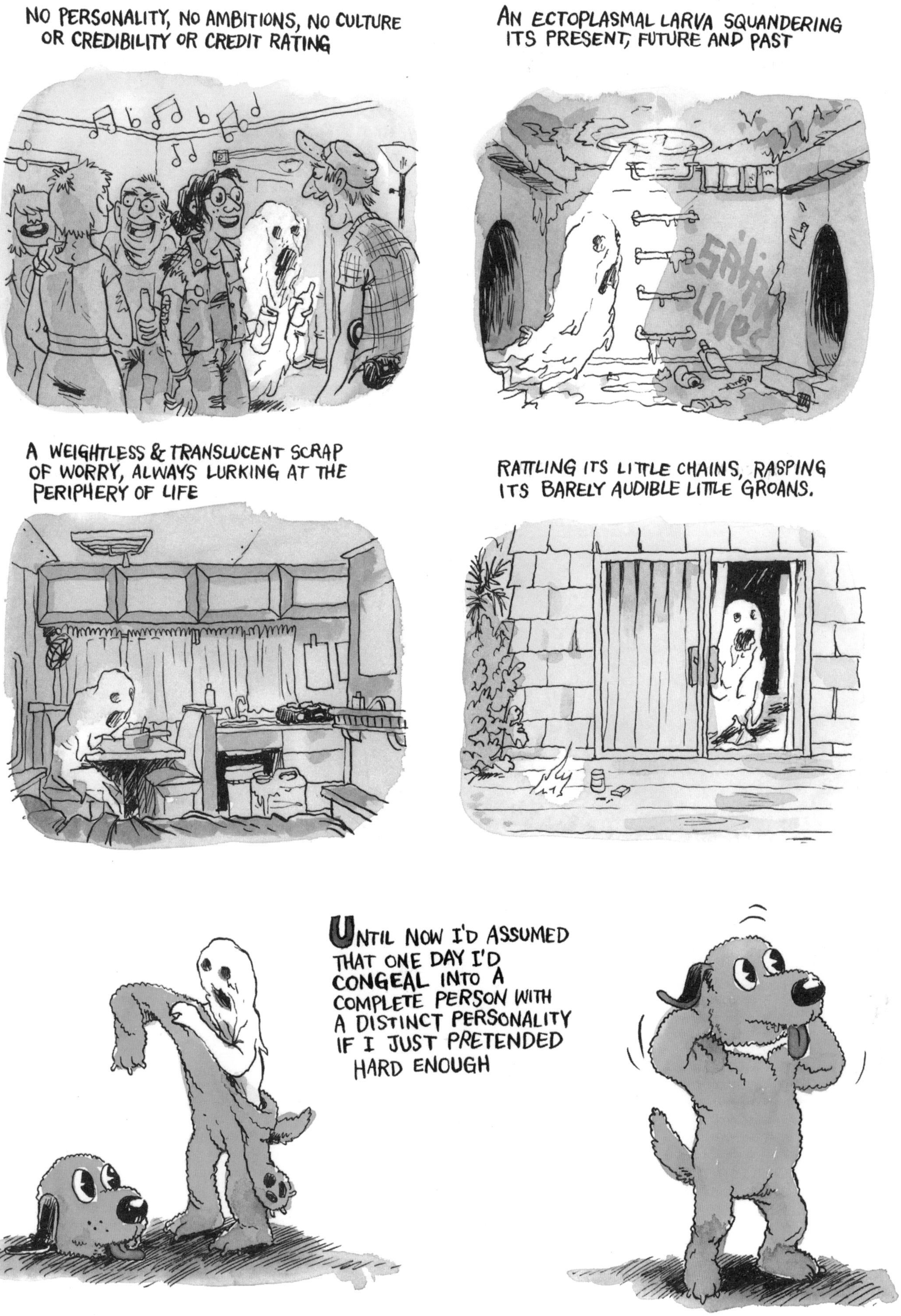
NO PERSONALITY, NO AMBITIONS, NO CULTURE OR CREDIBILITY OR CREDIT RATING
AN ECTOPLASMAL LARVA SQUANDERING ITS PRESENT, FUTURE AND PAST
A WEIGHTLESS & TRANSLUCENT SCRAP OF WORRY, ALWAYS LURKING AT THE PERIPHERY OF LIFE
RATTLING ITS LITTLE CHAINS, RASPING ITS BARELY AUDIBLE LITTLE GROANS.
UNTIL NOW I'D ASSUMED THAT ONE DAY I'D CONGEAL INTO A COMPLETE PERSON WITH A DISTINCT PERSONALITY IF I JUST PRETENDED HARD ENOUGH

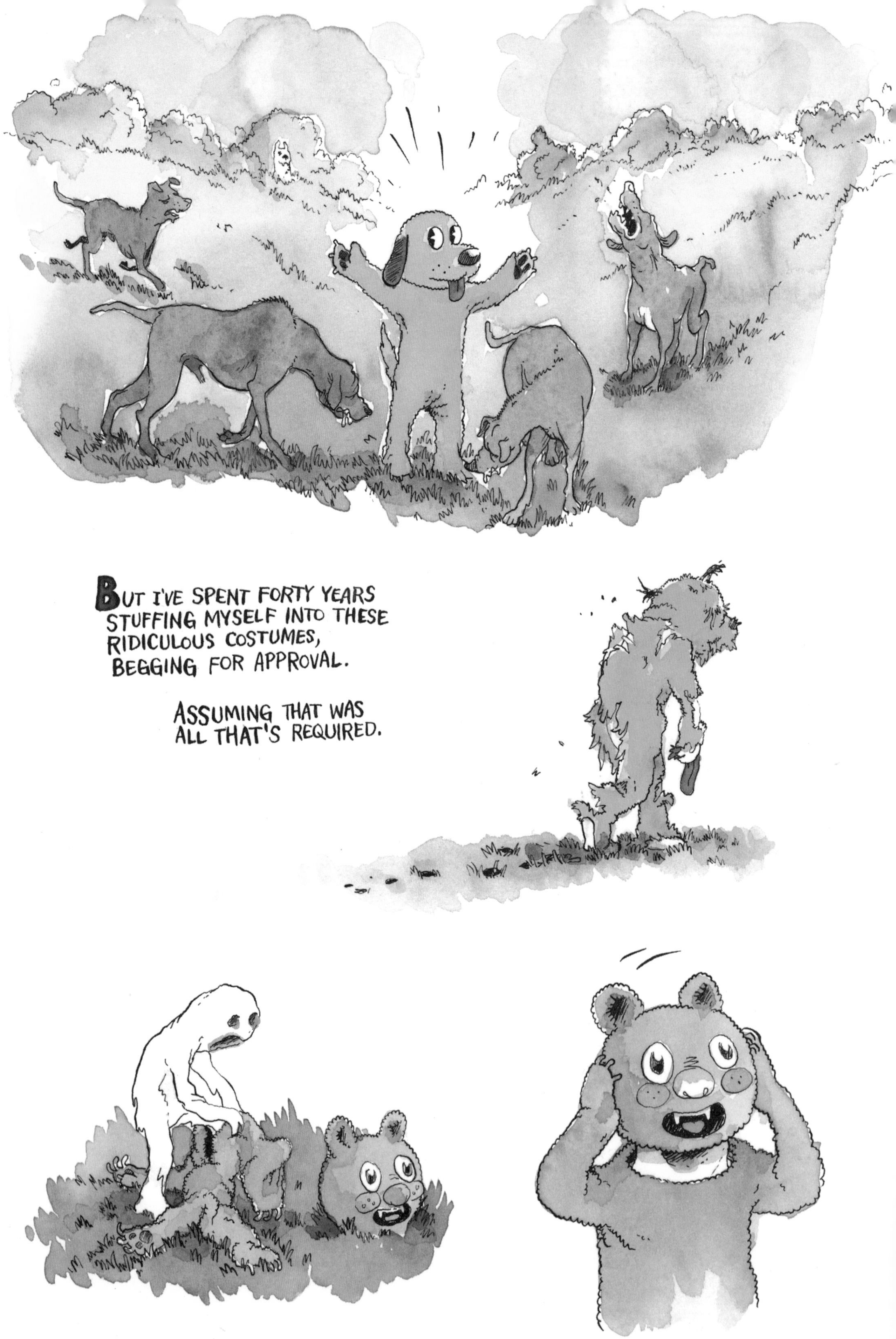
BUT I'VE SPENT FORTY YEARS STUFFING MYSELF INTO THESE RIDICULOUS COSTUMES, BEGGING FOR APPROVAL.
ASSUMING THAT WAS ALL THAT'S REQUIRED.

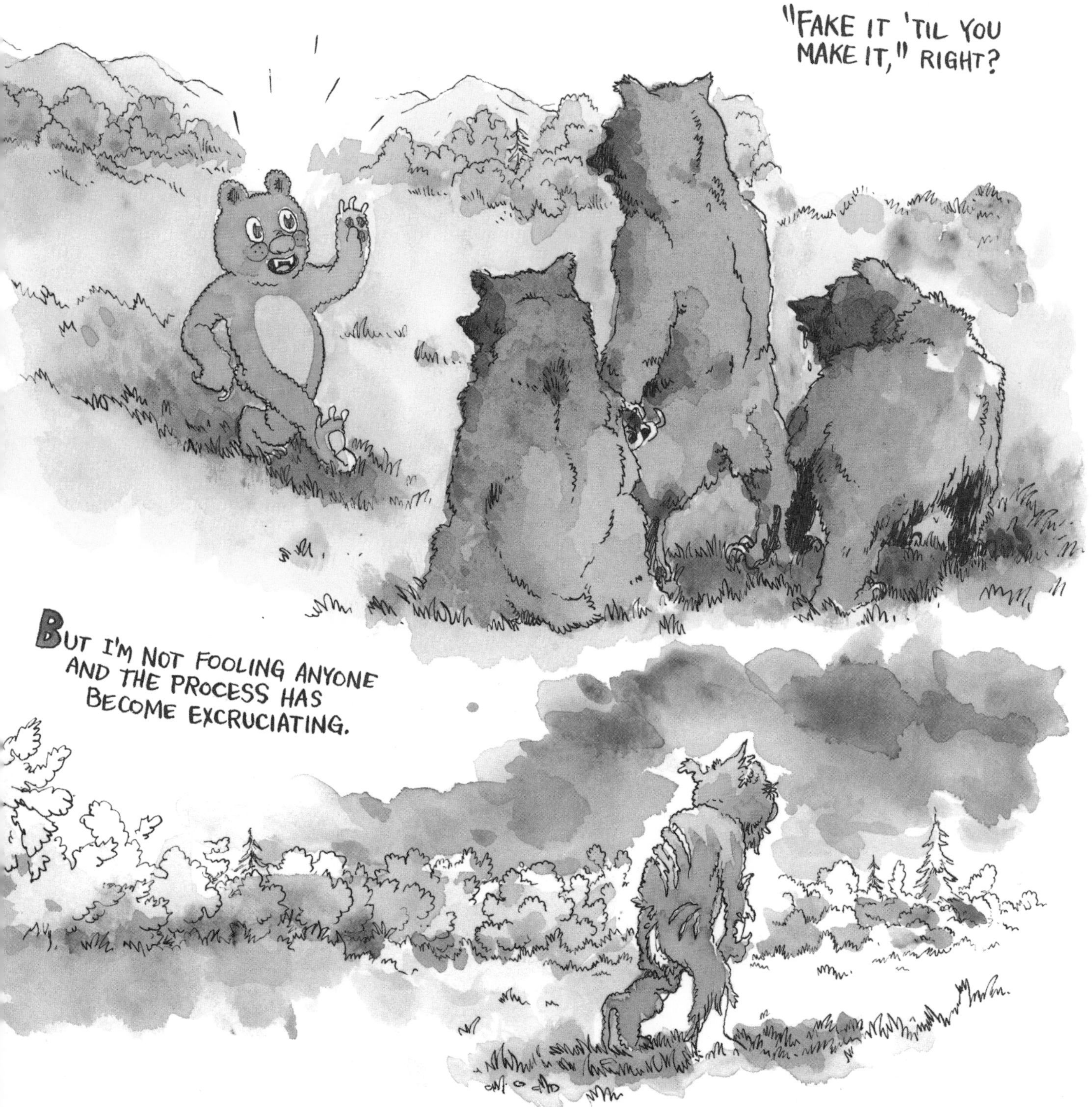
"FAKE IT 'TIL YOU MAKE IT," RIGHT?
BUT I'M NOT FOOLING ANYONE AND THE PROCESS HAS BECOME EXCRUCIATING.

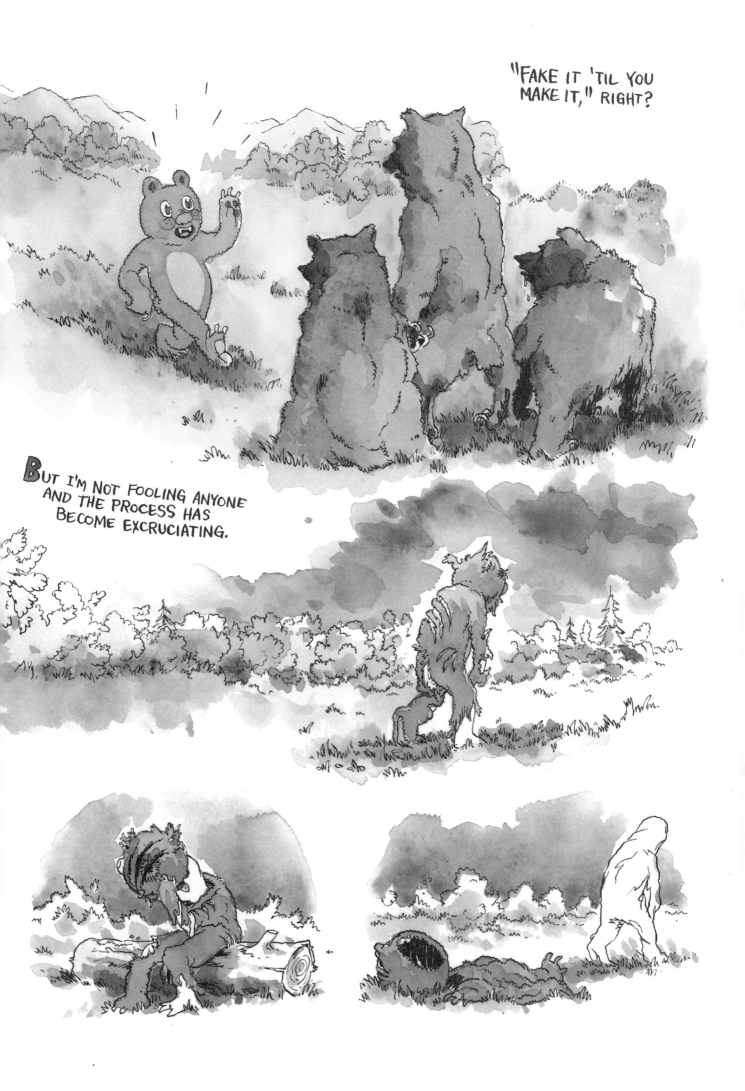

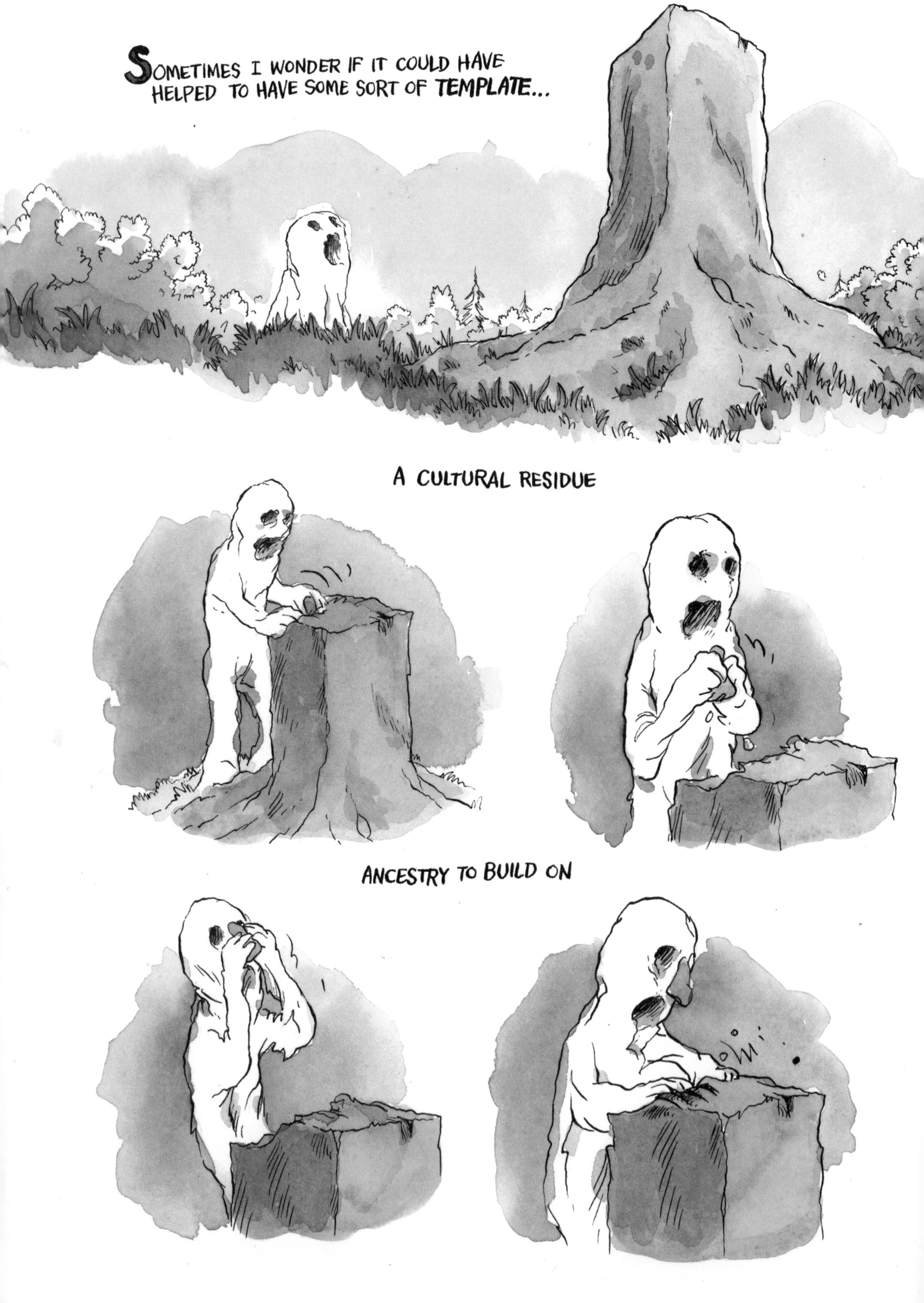
SOMETIMES I WONDER IF IT COULD HAVE HELPED TO HAVE SOME SORT OF TEMPLATE...
A CULTURAL RESIDUE
ANCESTRY TO BUILD ON

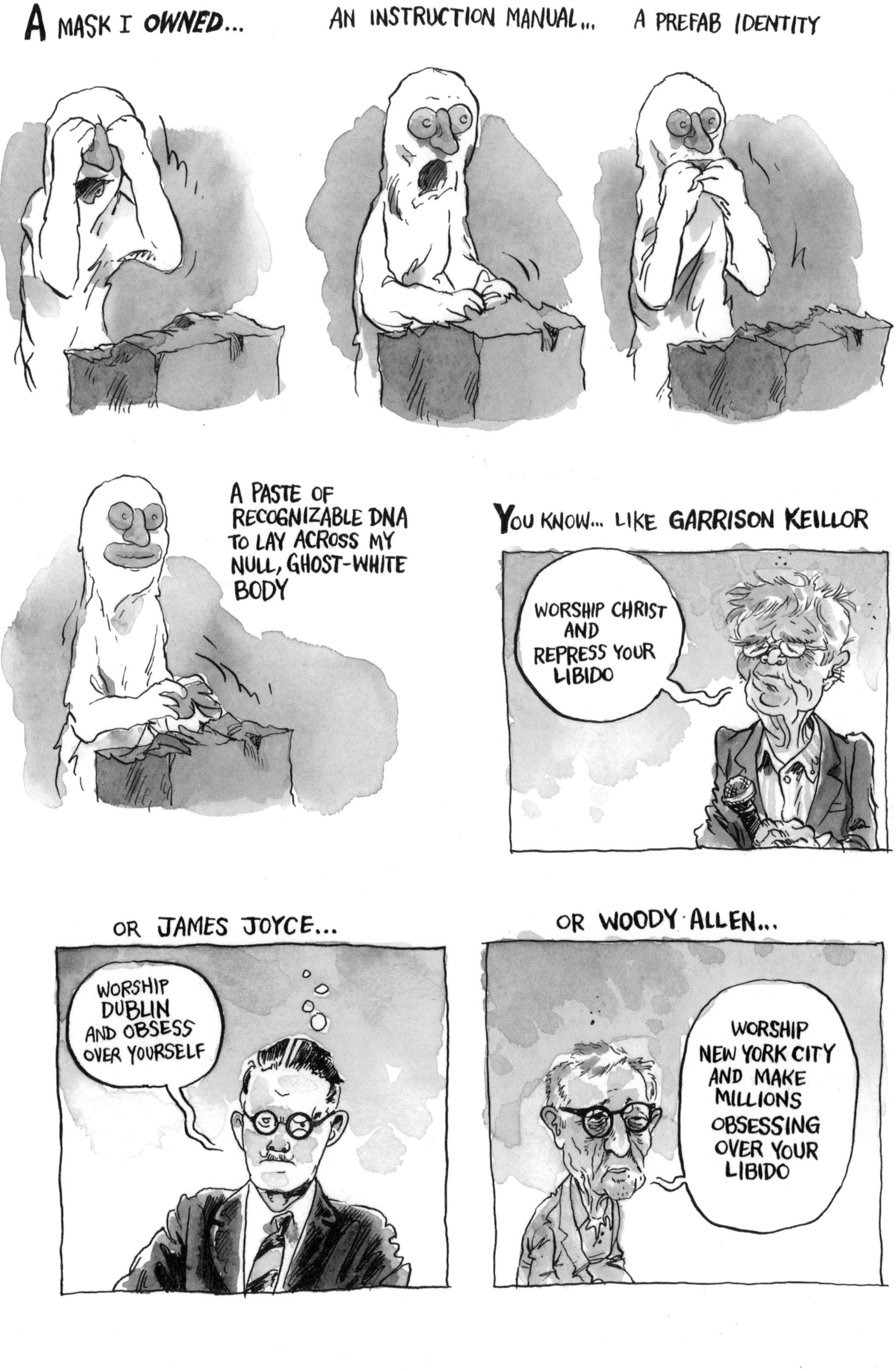

A MASK I OWNED...
AN INSTRUCTION MANUAL...
A PREFAB IDENTITY
A PASTE OF RECOGNIZABLE DNA TO LAY ACROSS MY NULL, GHOST-WHITE BODY
YOU KNOW... LIKE GARRISON KEILLOR
WORSHIP CHRIST AND REPRESS YOUR LIBIDO
OR JAMES JOYCE...
WORSHIP DUBLIN AND OBSESS OVER YOURSELF
OR WOODY ALLEN...
WORSHIP NEW YORK CITY AND MAKE MILLIONS OBSESSING OVER YOUR LIBIDO

BUT THAT'S JUST THE WHINING LAMENT OF ANOTHER PAMPERED WHITE AMERICAN GOY, ROMANTICIZING THE "SOUL" OF THE "OTHER," AFTER 500 YEARS OF GENOCIDE AND SLAVE-DRIVING HAS WITHERED HIS OWN AWAY

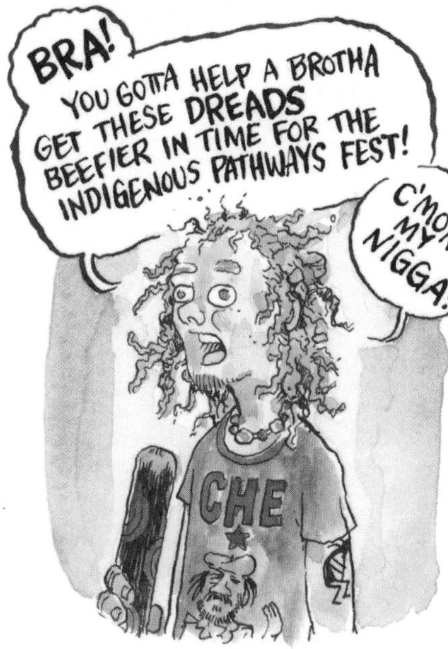
BRA! YOU GOTTA HELP A BROTHA GET THESE DREADS BEEFIER IN TIME FOR THE INDIGENOUS PATHWAYS FEST!
C'MON MY NIGGA!
CHE

THE CLOSEST THING I'VE GOT TO A REPRESENTATIVE OF MY "HERITAGE" IN POPULAR CULTURE IS PROBABLY **DAVID ALLEN COE...**

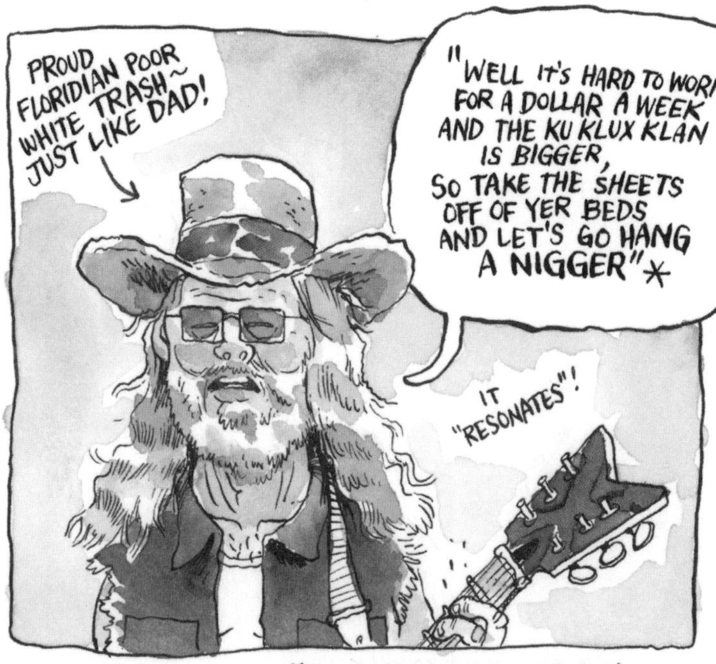
PROUD FLORIDIAN POOR WHITE TRASH~ JUST LIKE DAD!
"WELL IT'S HARD TO WORK FOR A DOLLAR A WEEK AND THE KU KLUX KLAN IS BIGGER, SO TAKE THE SHEETS OFF OF YER BEDS AND LET'S GO HANG A NIGGER"*
IT "RESONATES"!

*LYRICS FROM ACTUAL D.A.C. SONG

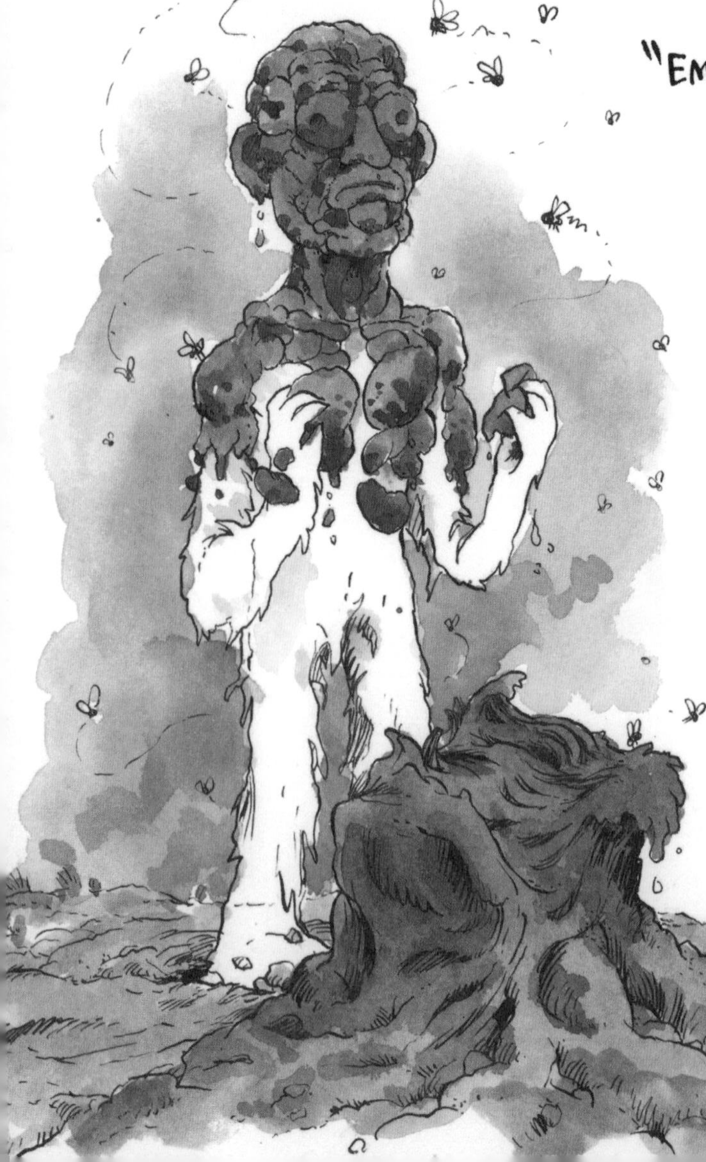

"EMBRACING MY HERITAGE" IS LIKE COVERING MYSELF IN SHIT

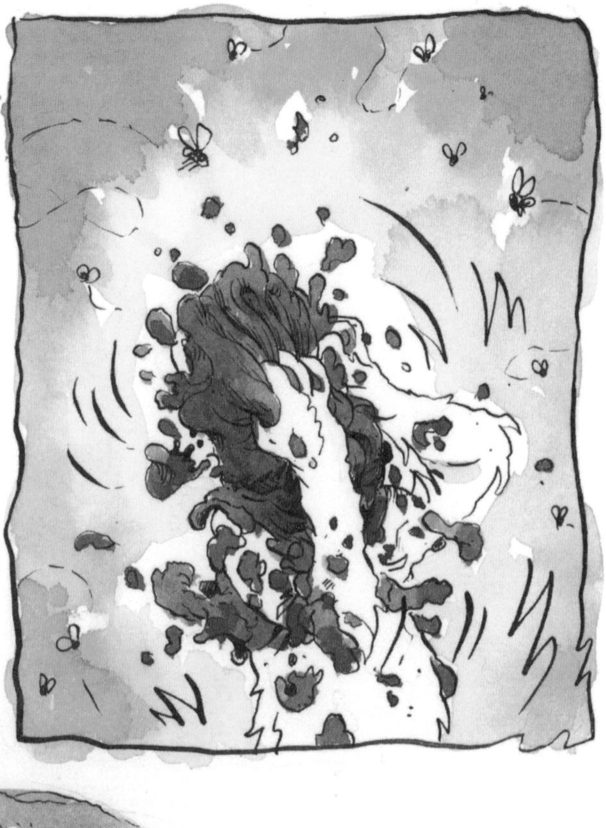

PLEASE DON'T MISUNDERSTAND ME.

I'M *EXTREMELY* GRATEFUL FOR THE JACKPOT OF PRIVILEGE FATE GRANTED ME WHEN I WAS BORN A **WHITE, ABLE, SANE, MIDDLE-CLASS, CISGENDERED MALE** IN THE "FIRST WORLD" AT THE END OF THE **20th CENTURY...**

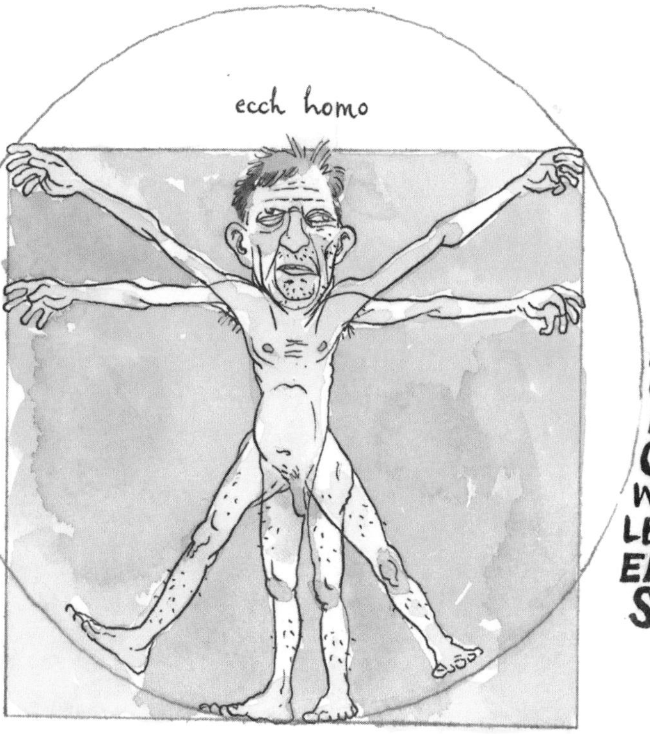
ecch homo

...EVEN THOUGH ALL THAT PRIVILEGE COMES BUNDLED WITH A HIGHLY CONDITIONAL **COMPLICITY** IN THE WHITE MALE'S RICH LEGACY OF **VIOLENCE, ENTITLEMENT,** AND **SOCIOPATHIC GREED...**

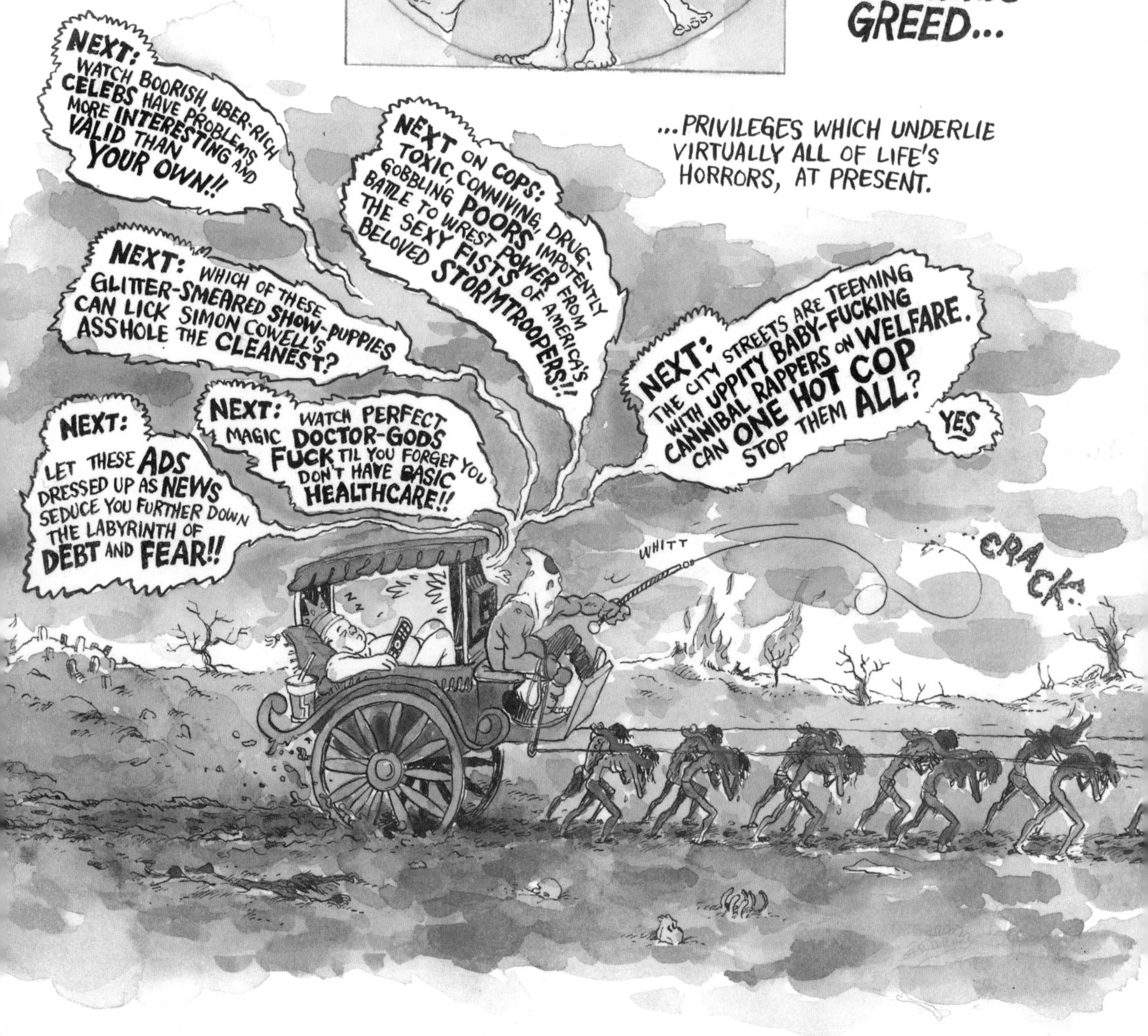
...PRIVILEGES WHICH UNDERLIE VIRTUALLY ALL OF LIFE'S HORRORS, AT PRESENT.
NEXT: WATCH BOORISH, UBER-RICH CELEBS HAVE PROBLEMS MORE INTERESTING AND VALID THAN YOUR OWN!!
NEXT ON COPS: TOXIC, CONNIVING, DRUG-GOBBLING POORS IMPOTENTLY BATTLE TO WREST POWER FROM THE SEXY FISTS OF AMERICA'S BELOVED STORMTROOPERS!!
NEXT: WHICH OF THESE GLITTER-SMEARED SHOW-PUPPIES CAN LICK SIMON COWELL'S ASSHOLE THE CLEANEST?
NEXT: THE CITY STREETS ARE TEEMING WITH UPPITY BABY-FUCKING CANNIBAL RAPPERS ON WELFARE. CAN ONE HOT COP STOP THEM ALL?
YES
NEXT: LET THESE ADS DRESSED UP AS NEWS SEDUCE YOU FURTHER DOWN THE LABYRINTH OF DEBT AND FEAR!!
NEXT: WATCH PERFECT, MAGIC DOCTOR-GODS FUCK TIL YOU FORGET YOU DON'T HAVE BASIC HEALTHCARE!!
WHITT
CRACK

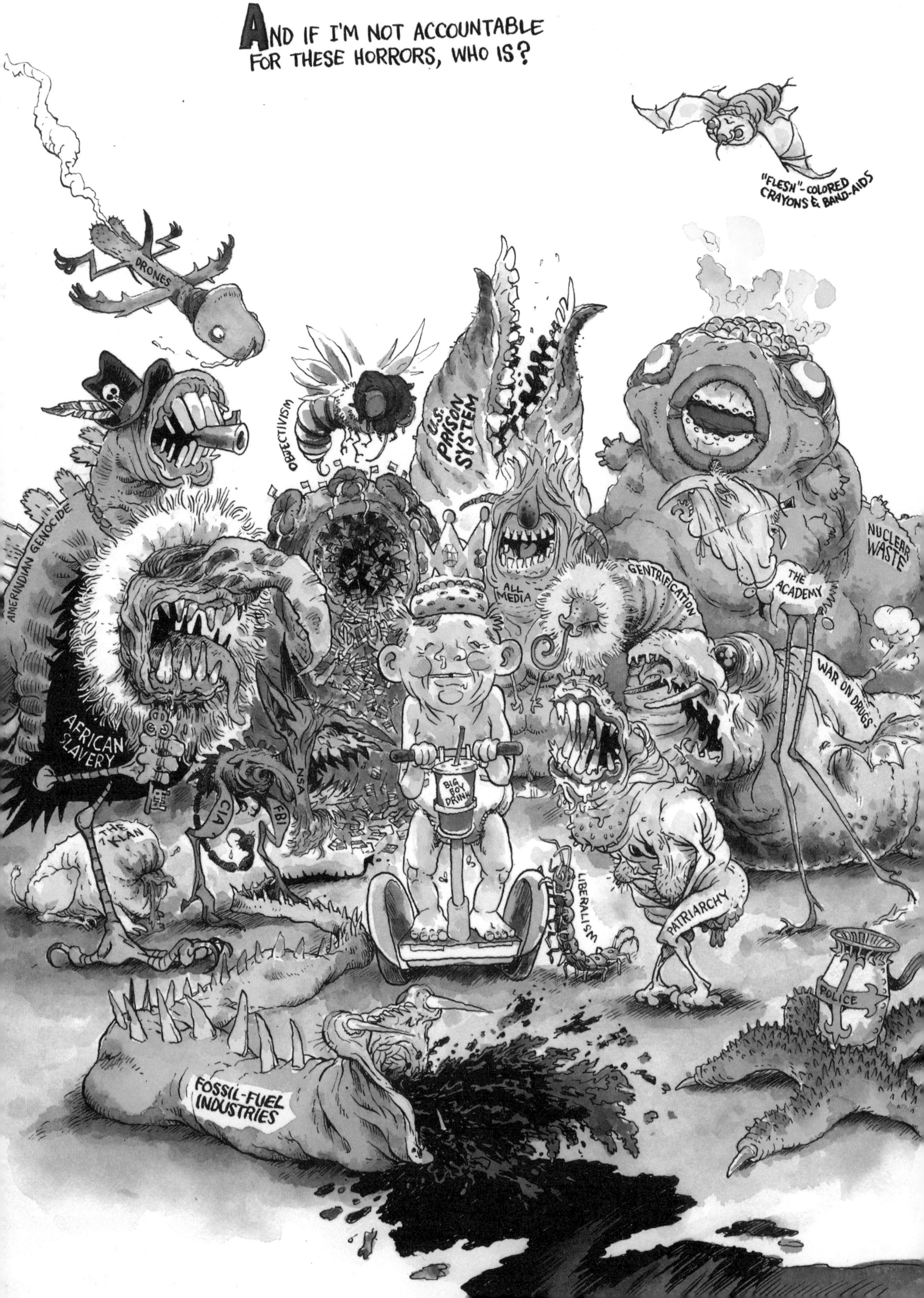
AND IF I'M NOT ACCOUNTABLE FOR THESE HORRORS, WHO IS?
"FLESH"-COLORED CRAYONS & BAND-AIDS
DRONES
OBJECTIVISM
U.S. PRISON SYSTEM
NUCLEAR WASTE
AMERINDIAN GENOCIDE
ALL MEDIA
GENTRIFICATION
THE ACADEMY
WAR ON DRUGS
AFRICAN SLAVERY
NSA
CIA
FBI
BIG BOY DRINK
THE KLAN
LIBERALISM
PATRIARCHY
POLICE
FOSSIL-FUEL INDUSTRIES

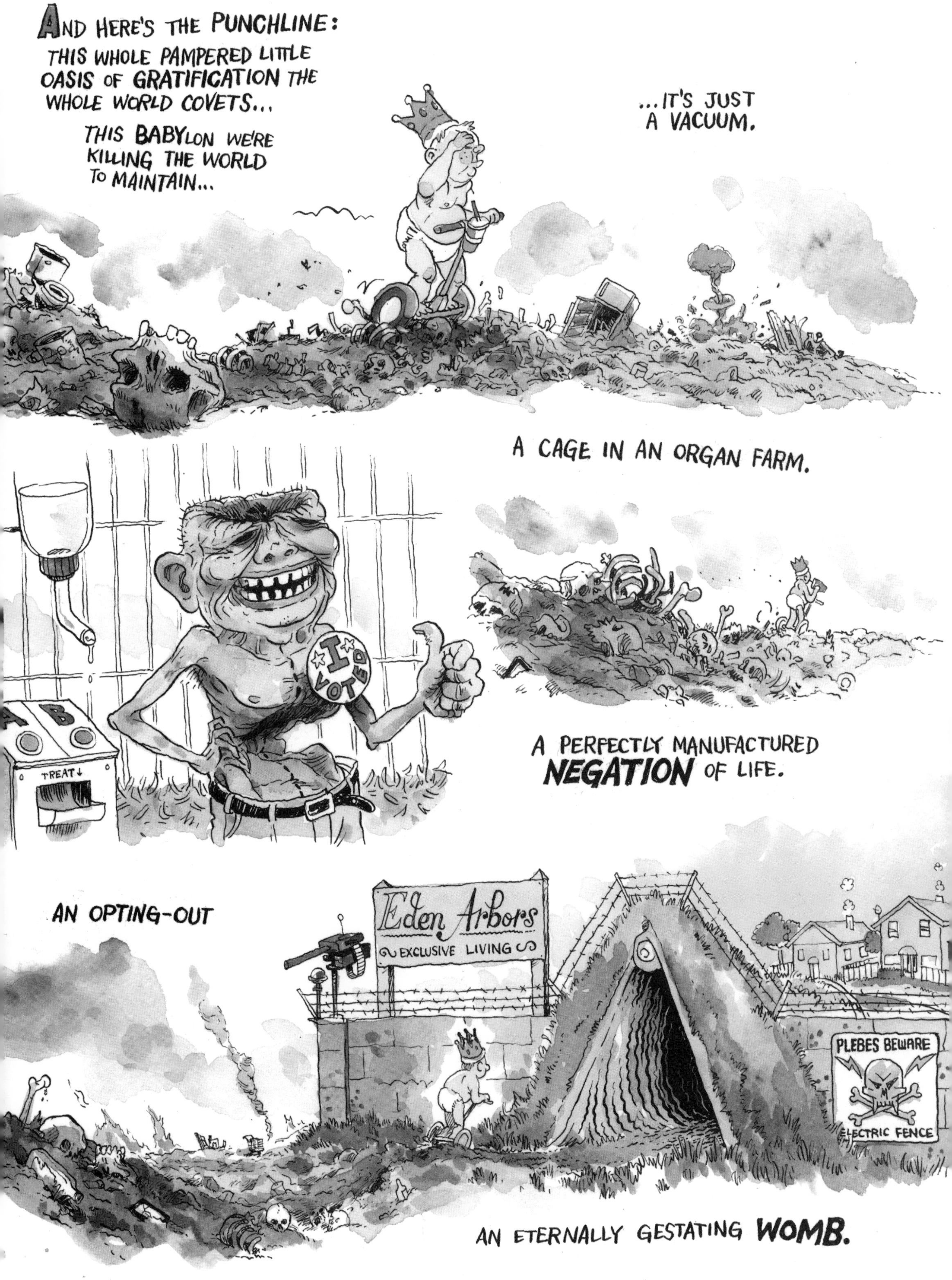
AND HERE'S THE PUNCHLINE:
THIS WHOLE PAMPERED LITTLE OASIS OF GRATIFICATION THE WHOLE WORLD COVETS...
THIS BABYLON WE'RE KILLING THE WORLD TO MAINTAIN...
...IT'S JUST A VACUUM.
A CAGE IN AN ORGAN FARM.
I VOTED
A
B
TREAT↓
A PERFECTLY MANUFACTURED NEGATION OF LIFE.
AN OPTING-OUT
Eden Arbors
EXCLUSIVE LIVING
PLEBES BEWARE
ELECTRIC FENCE
AN ETERNALLY GESTATING WOMB.

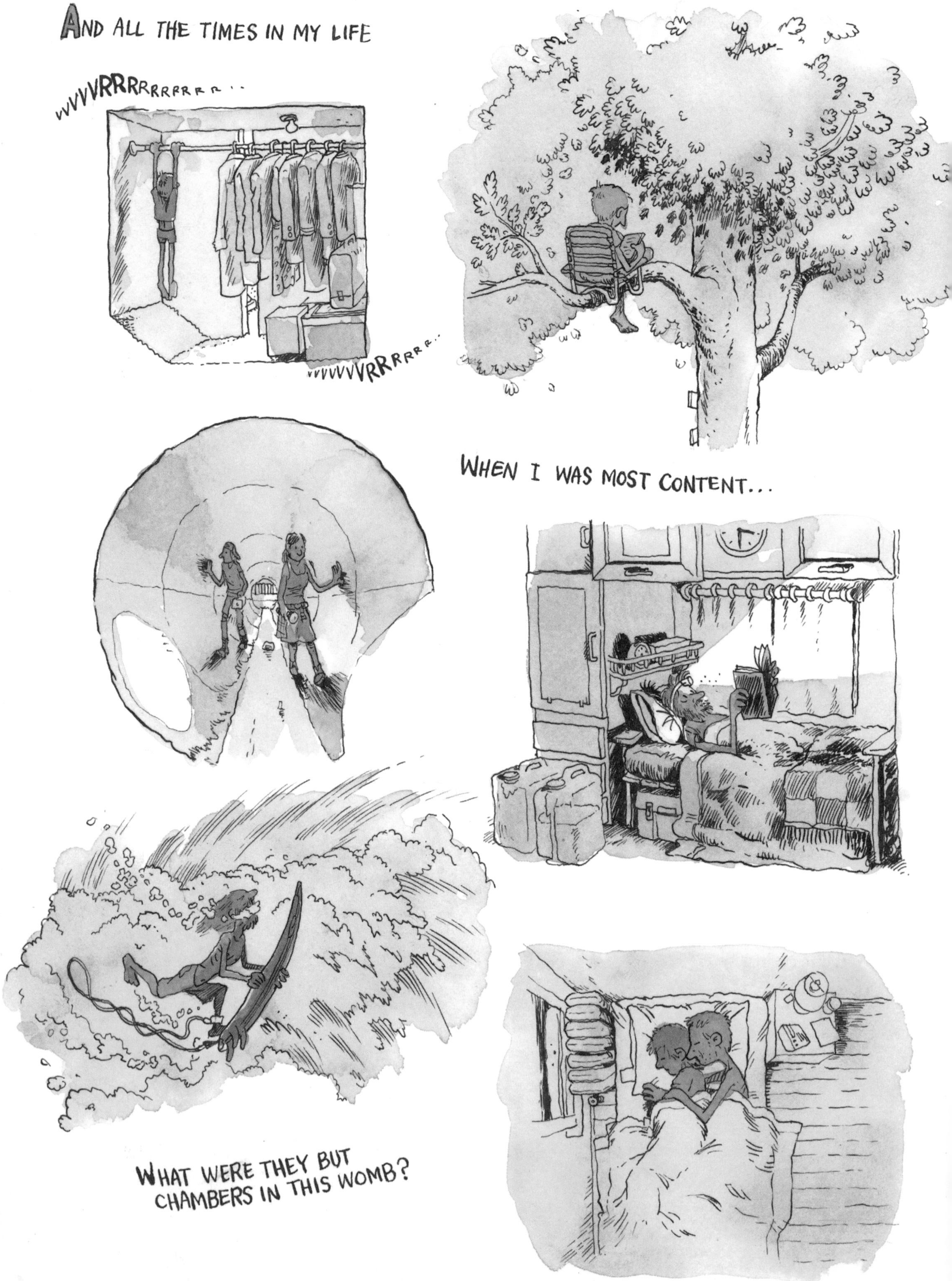
AND ALL THE TIMES IN MY LIFE
vvvvVRRRrrrrrrr . .
vvvvvvVRRrrrr . .
WHEN I WAS MOST CONTENT...
WHAT WERE THEY BUT
CHAMBERS IN THIS WOMB?

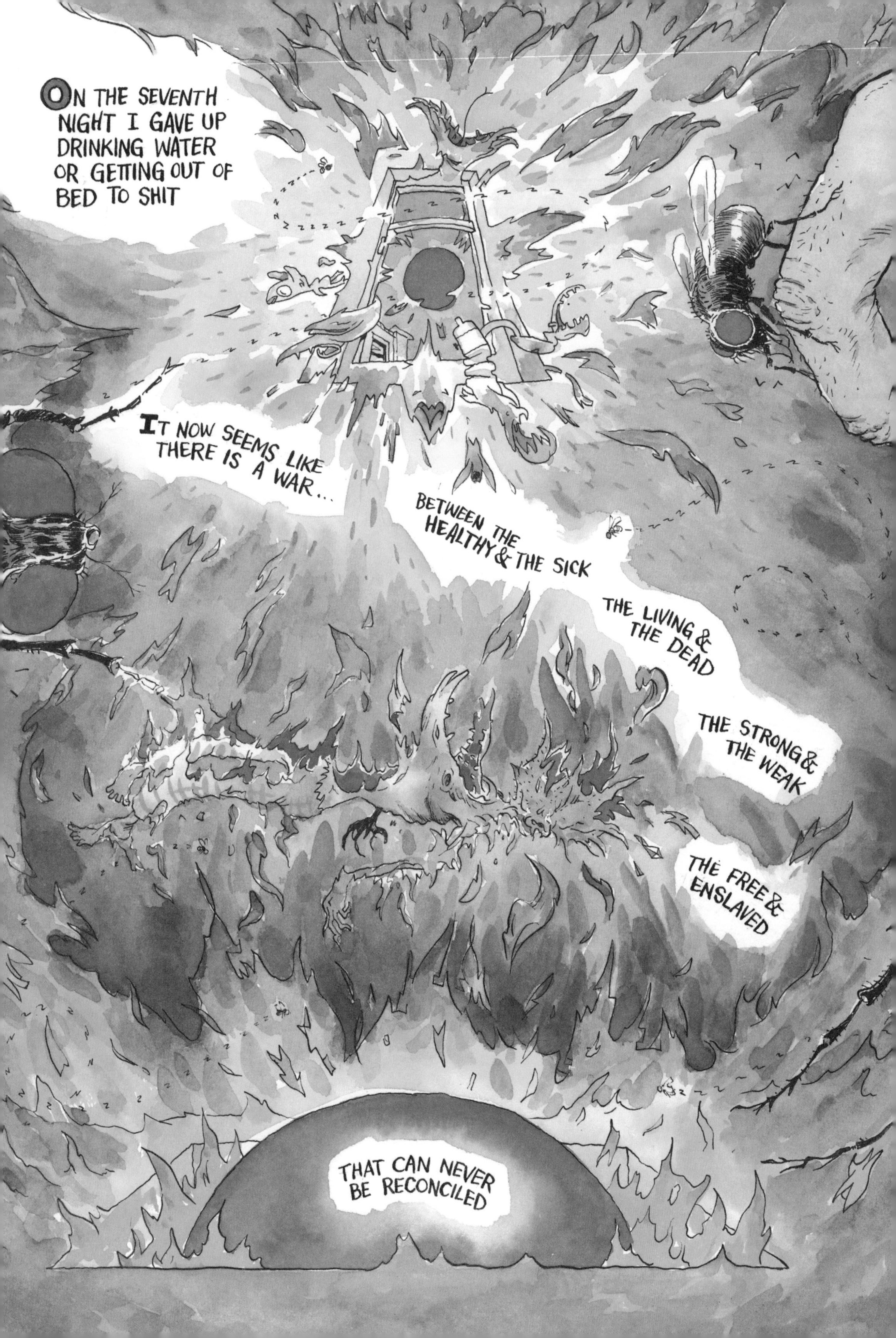
ON THE SEVENTH NIGHT I GAVE UP DRINKING WATER OR GETTING OUT OF BED TO SHIT
IT NOW SEEMS LIKE THERE IS A WAR...
BETWEEN THE HEALTHY & THE SICK
THE LIVING & THE DEAD
THE STRONG & THE WEAK
THE FREE & ENSLAVED
THAT CAN NEVER BE RECONCILED

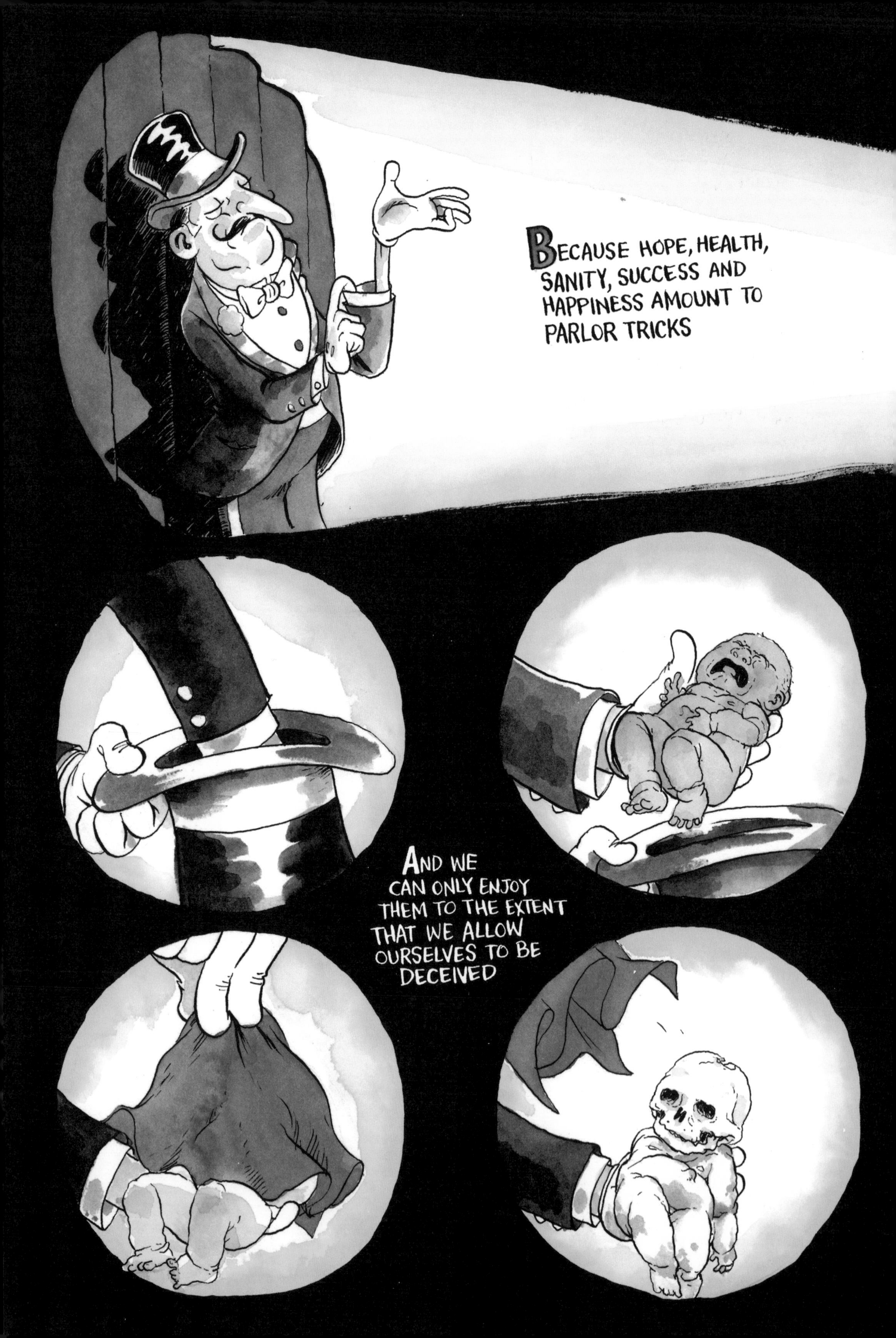
BECAUSE HOPE, HEALTH, SANITY, SUCCESS AND HAPPINESS AMOUNT TO PARLOR TRICKS
AND WE CAN ONLY ENJOY THEM TO THE EXTENT THAT WE ALLOW OURSELVES TO BE DECEIVED

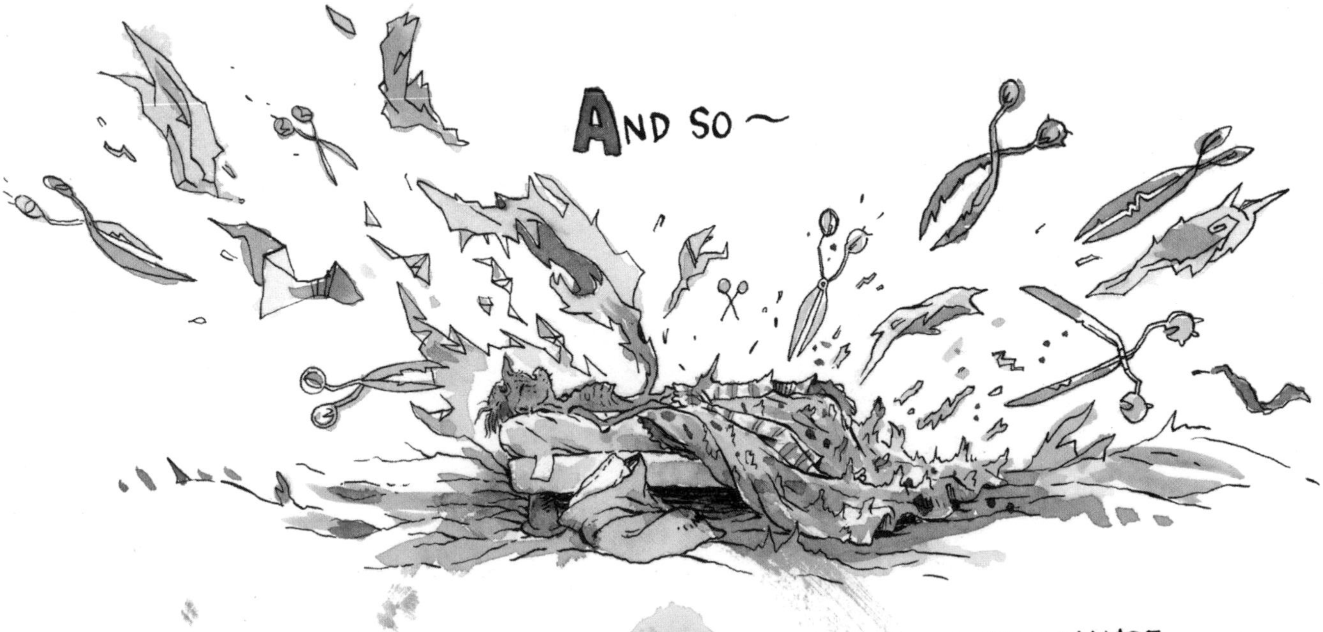
AND SO ~

IF MY WHOLE EXISTENCE WAS JUST A QUAINT LITTLE PERFORMANCE

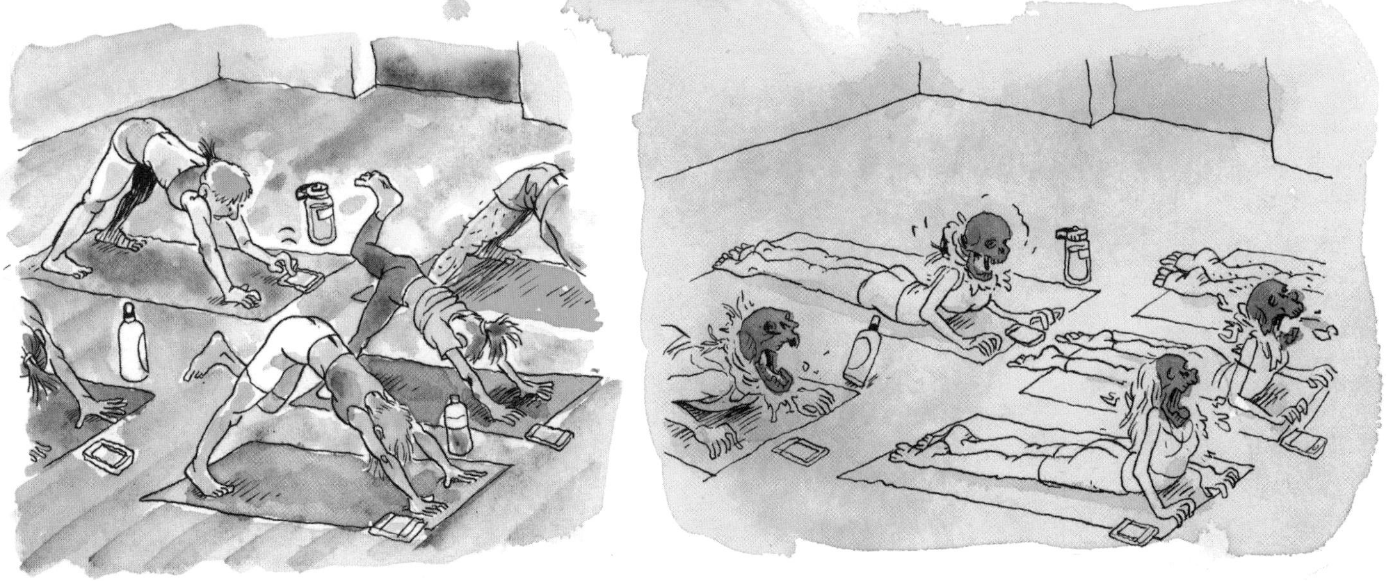

IF MY COMFORT AND SAFETY IS PREDICATED ON THE SUFFERING OF BILLIONS

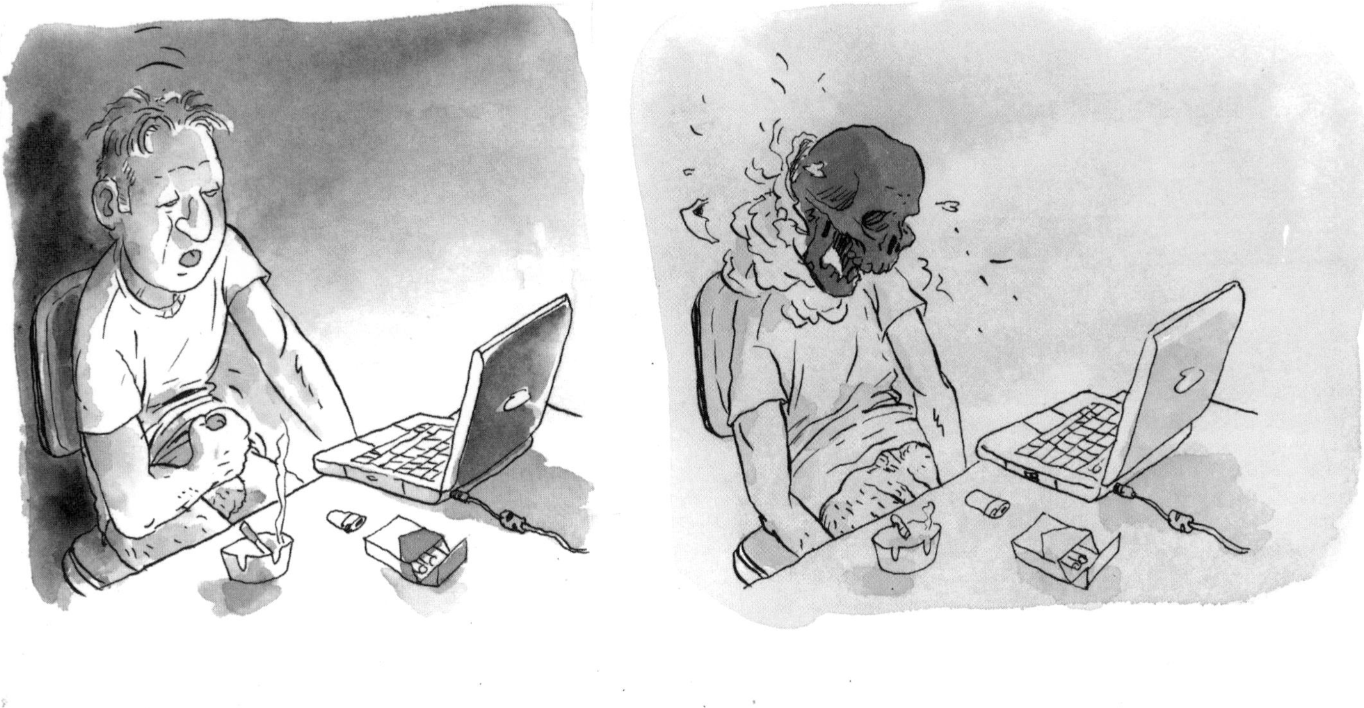

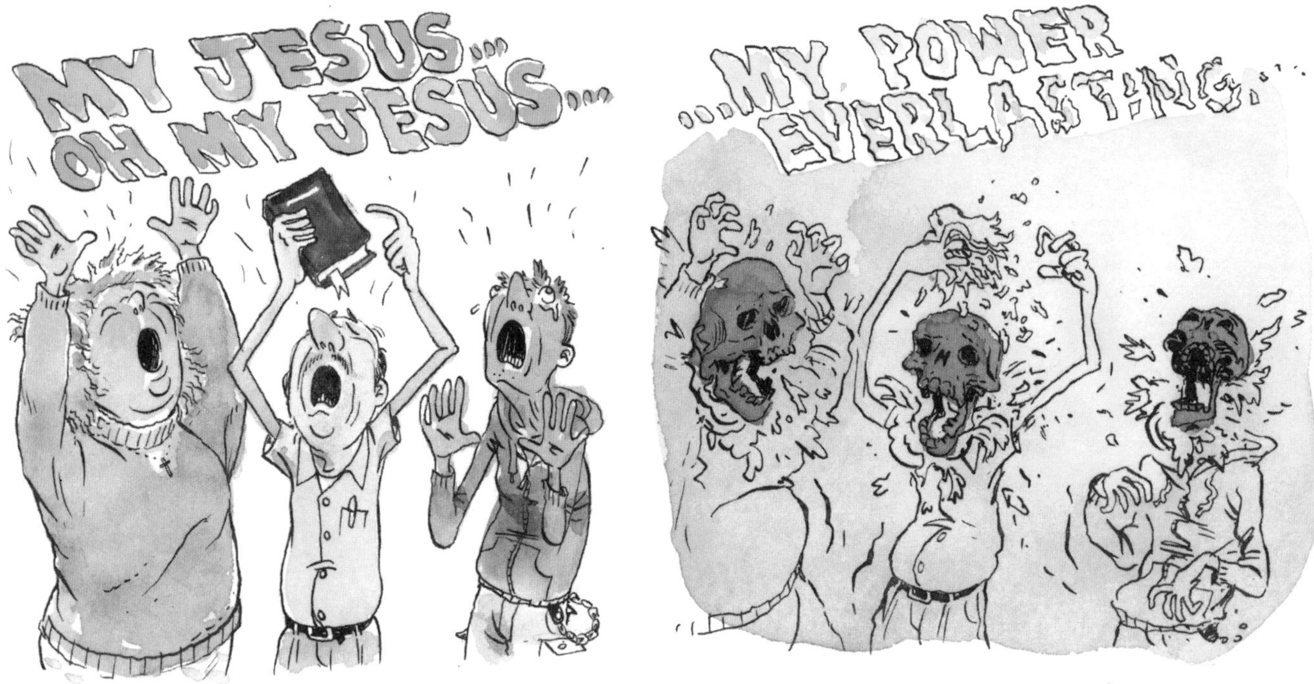
MY JESUS... OH MY JESUS...
...MY POWER EVERLASTING...

IF HAPPINESS DEMANDS THAT WE SHIELD OUR EYES TO TRUTH

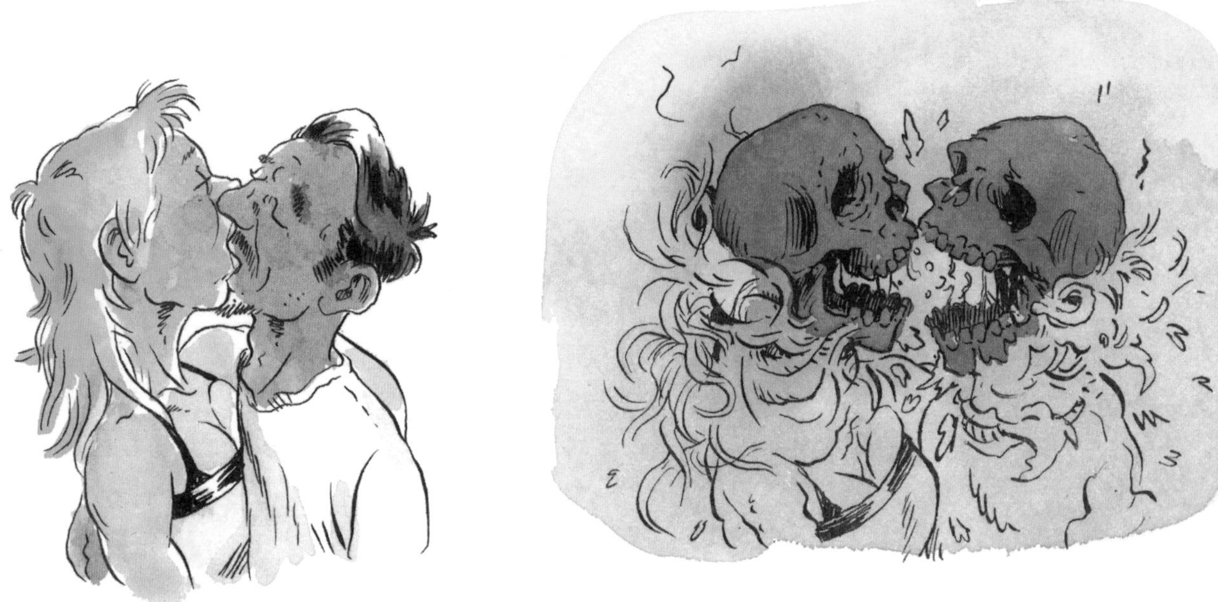

IF THE WHOLE WORLD IS A SPECK OF ASH IN AN INFINITE STERILE ABYSS

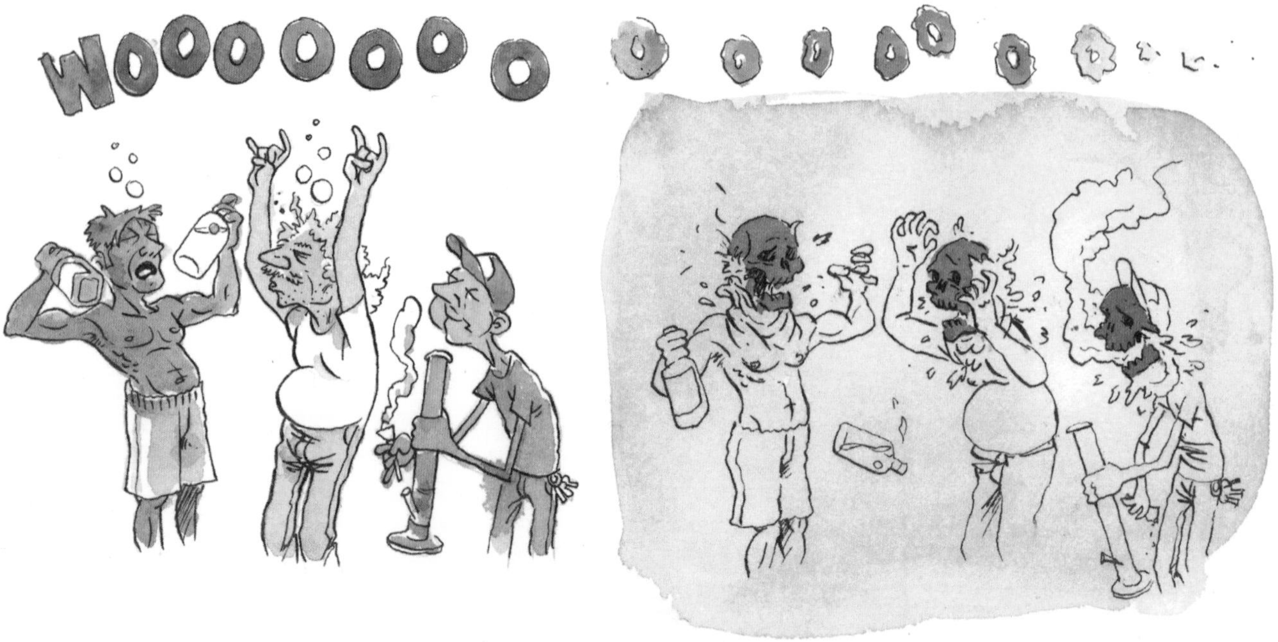
WOOOOOOO

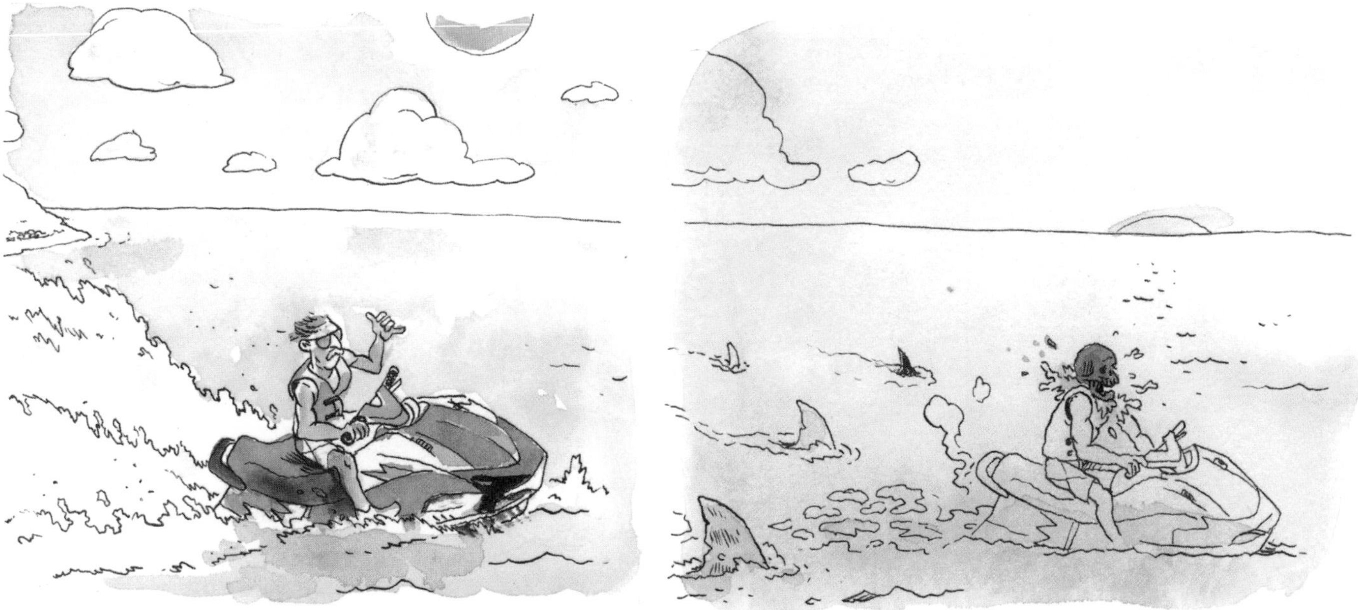

IF IT'S CERTAIN OUR PRESENCE IS A BLIGHT ON A FRAGILE PLANET

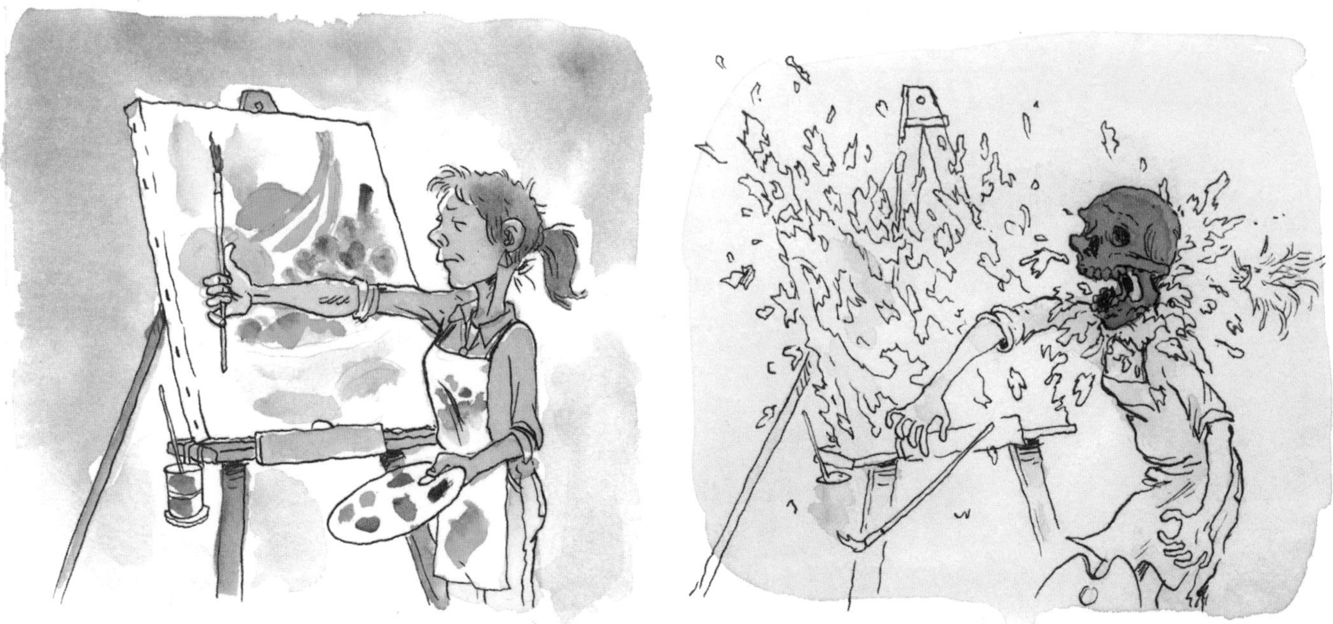

IF ALL WISDOM LEADS US ONLY INTO A PRIVATE HELL

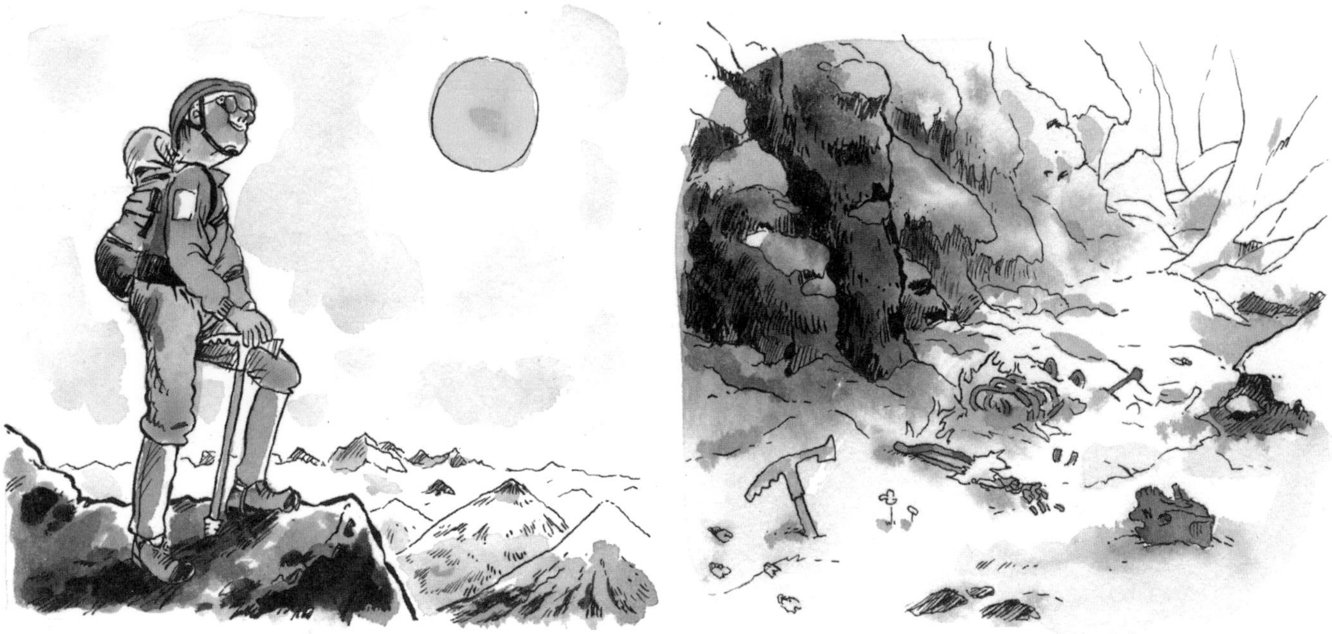

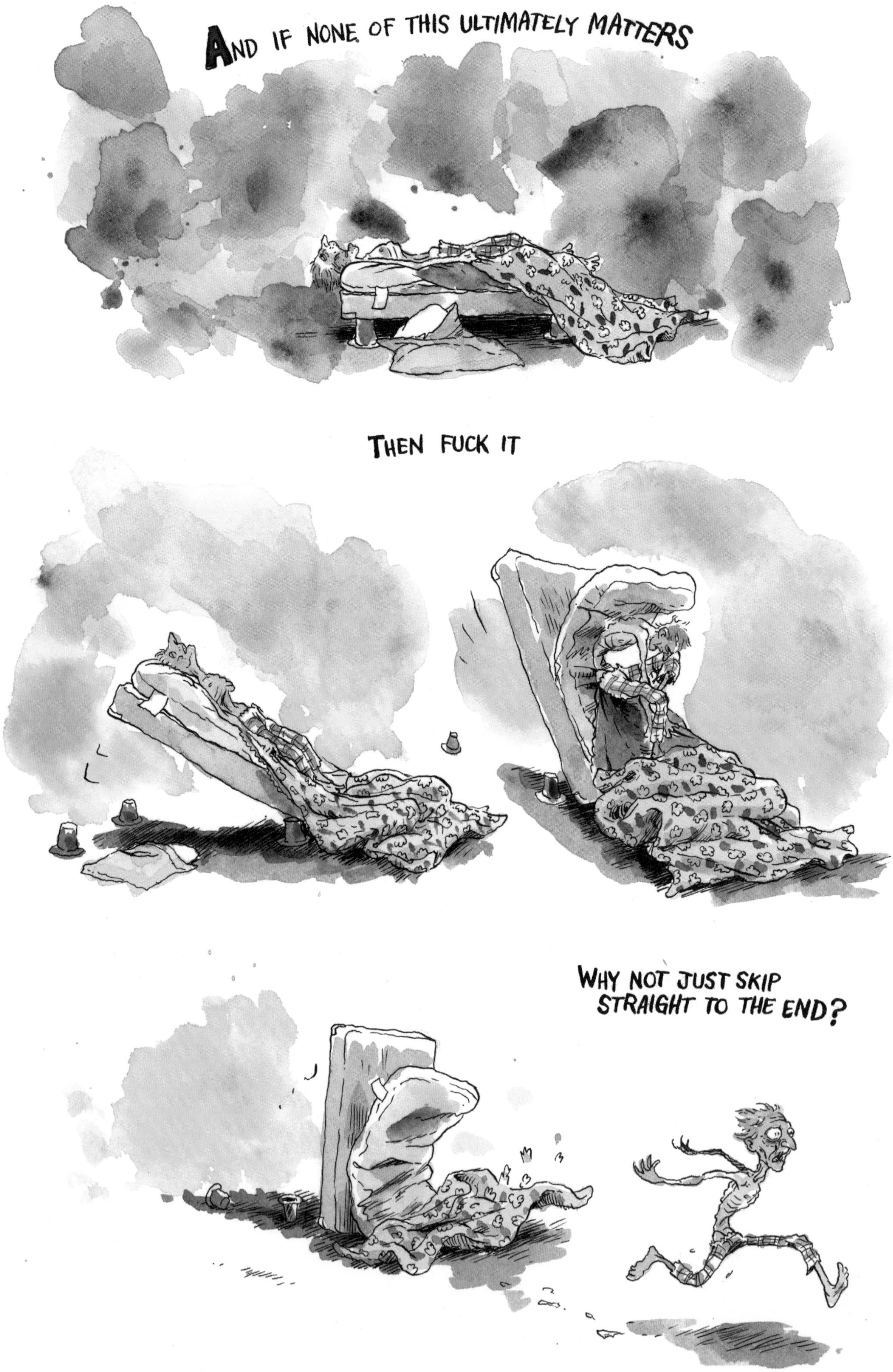
AND IF NONE OF THIS ULTIMATELY MATTERS
THEN FUCK IT
WHY NOT JUST SKIP STRAIGHT TO THE END?

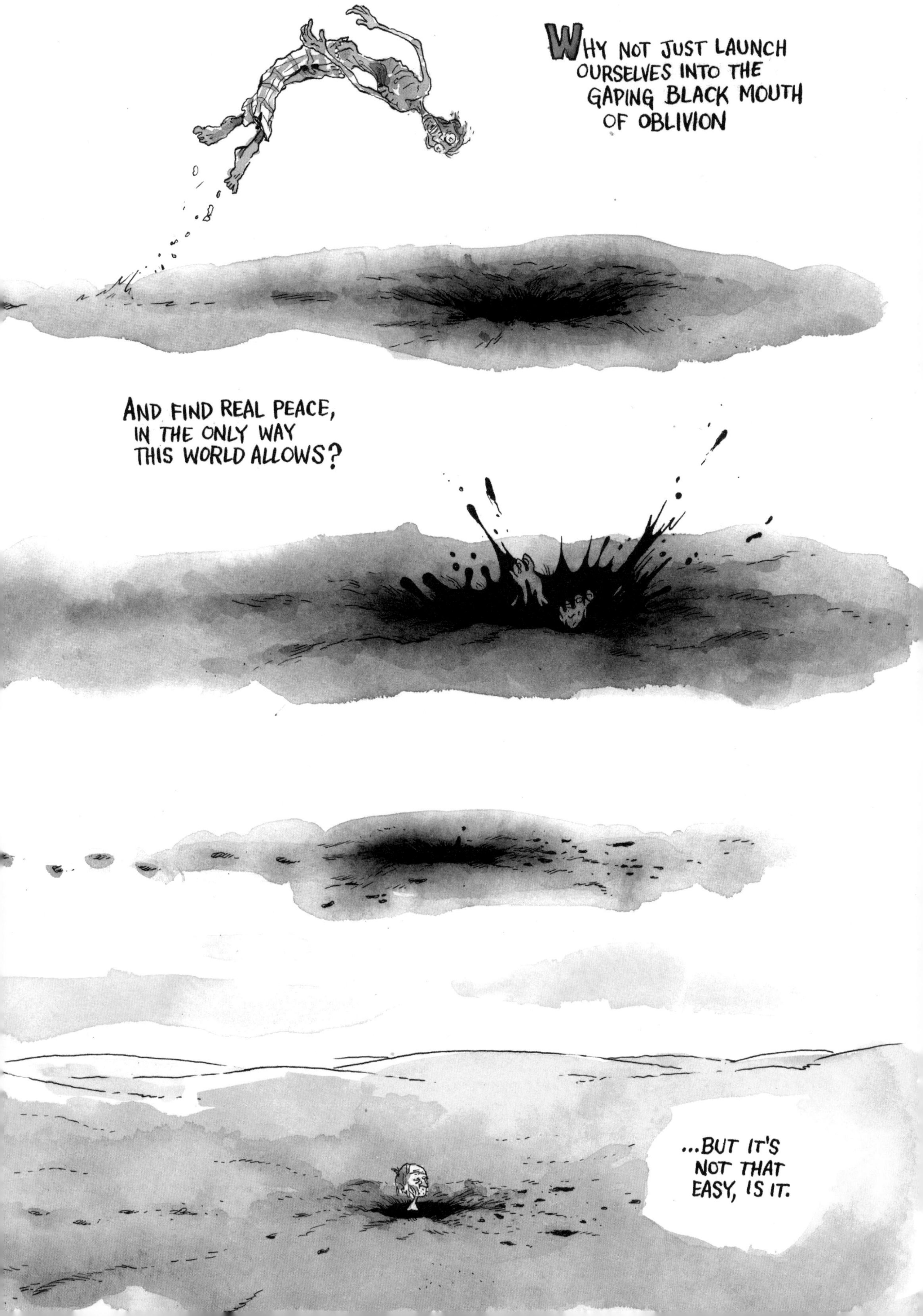
WHY NOT JUST LAUNCH OURSELVES INTO THE GAPING BLACK MOUTH OF OBLIVION
AND FIND REAL PEACE, IN THE ONLY WAY THIS WORLD ALLOWS?
...BUT IT'S NOT THAT EASY, IS IT.

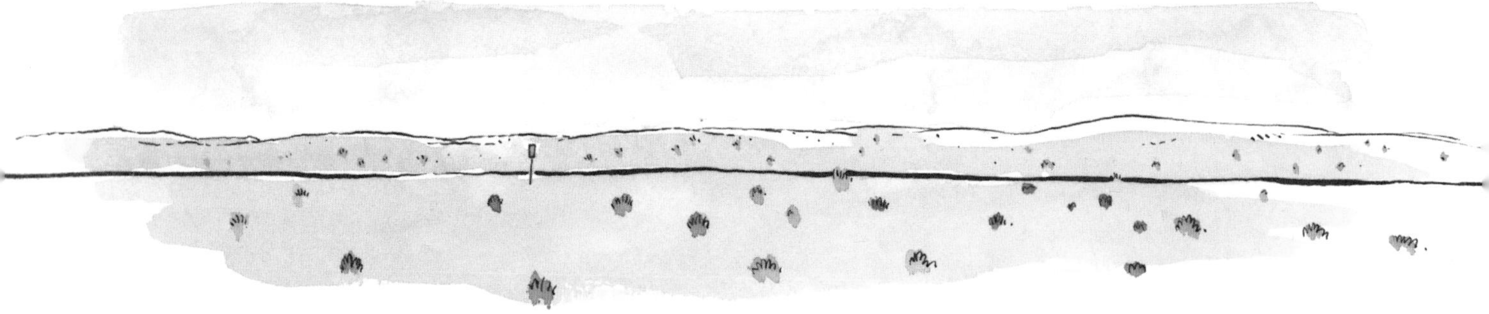

WE'RE IMPRISONED IN BODIES THAT STRUGGLE FOR LIFE

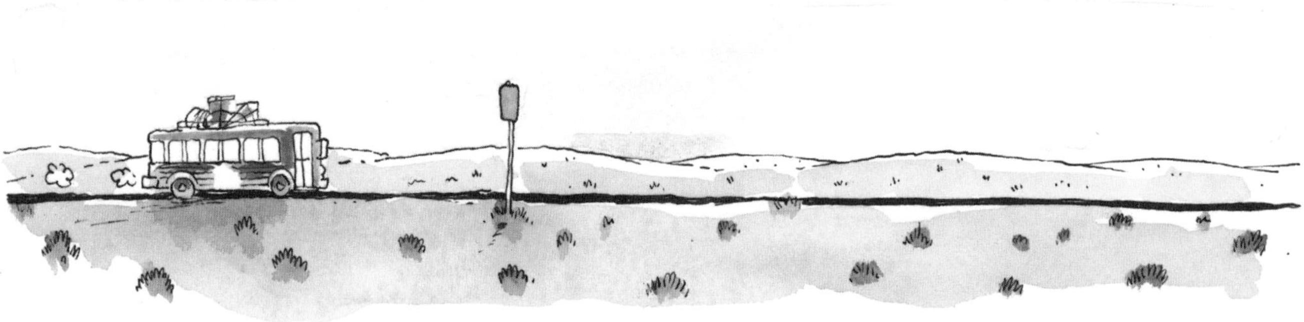

HOPE GESTATES IN US LIKE A TUMOR

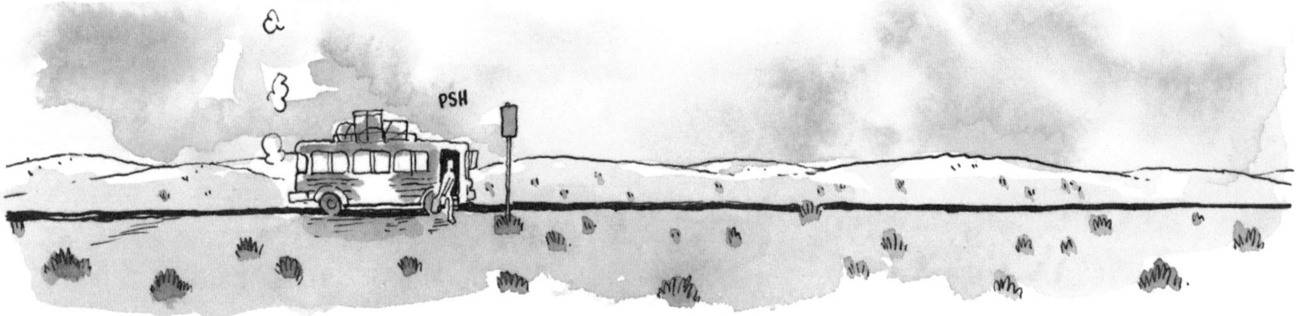
PSH

OR A NIGHTMARE IN OUR SLEEPING BRAINS

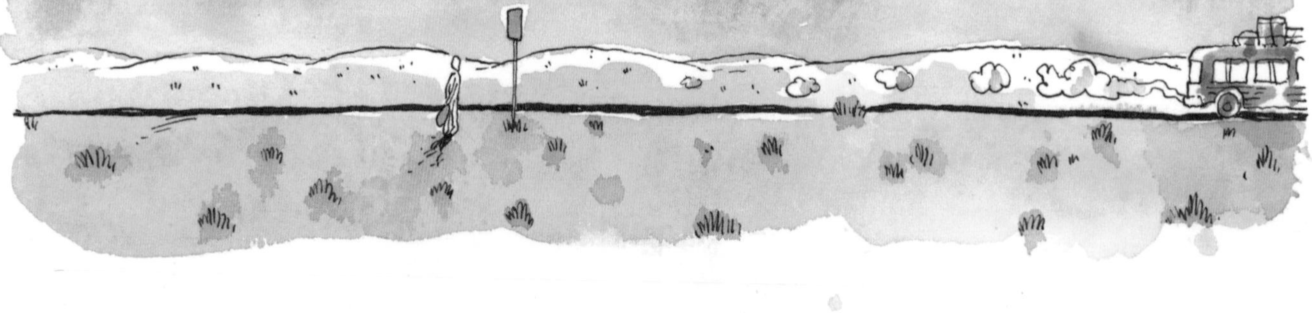

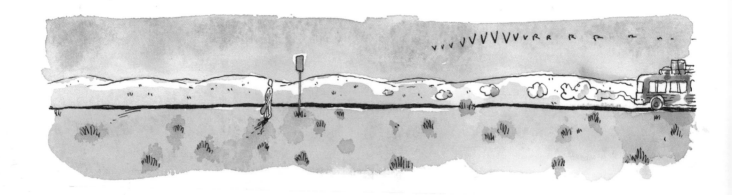

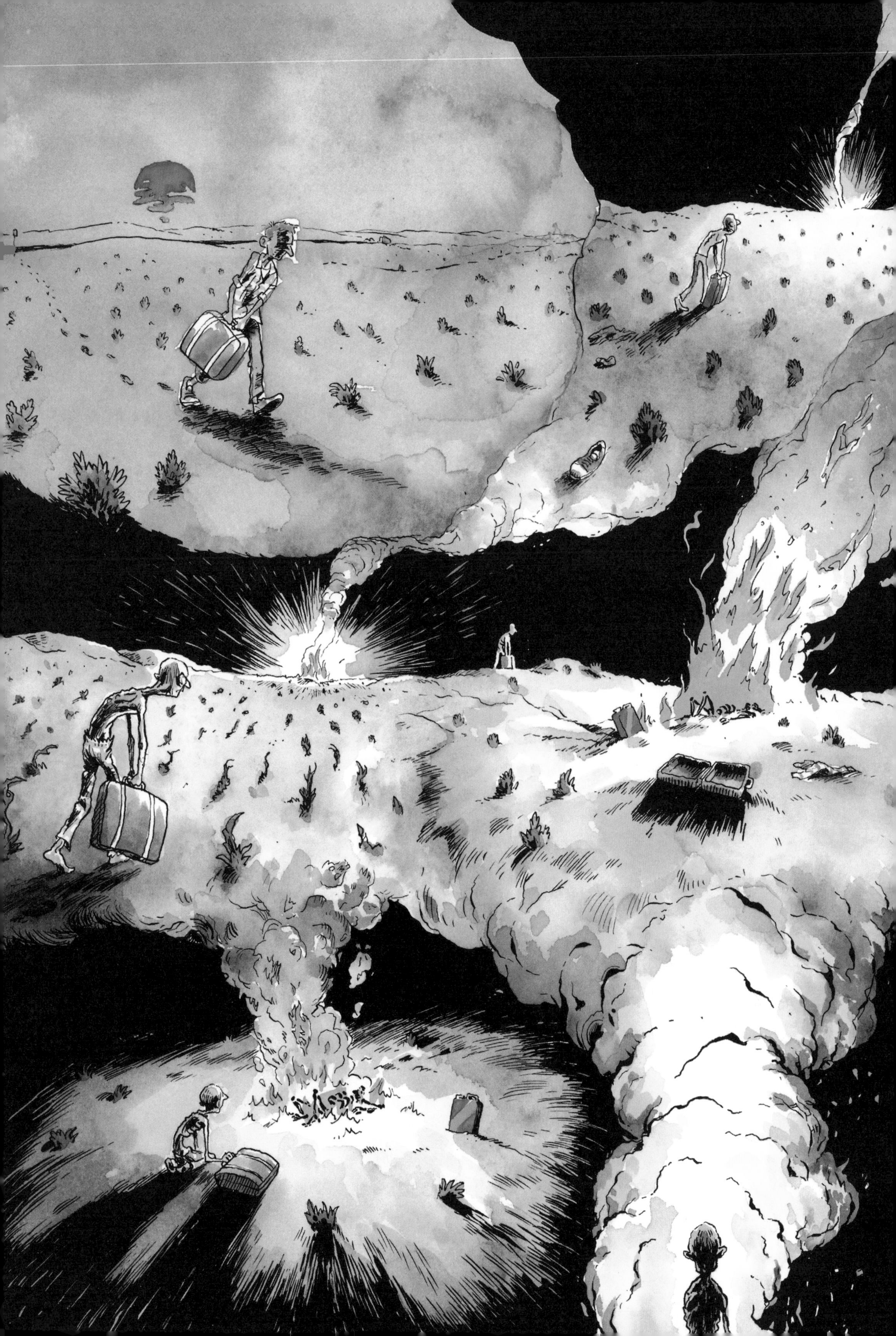

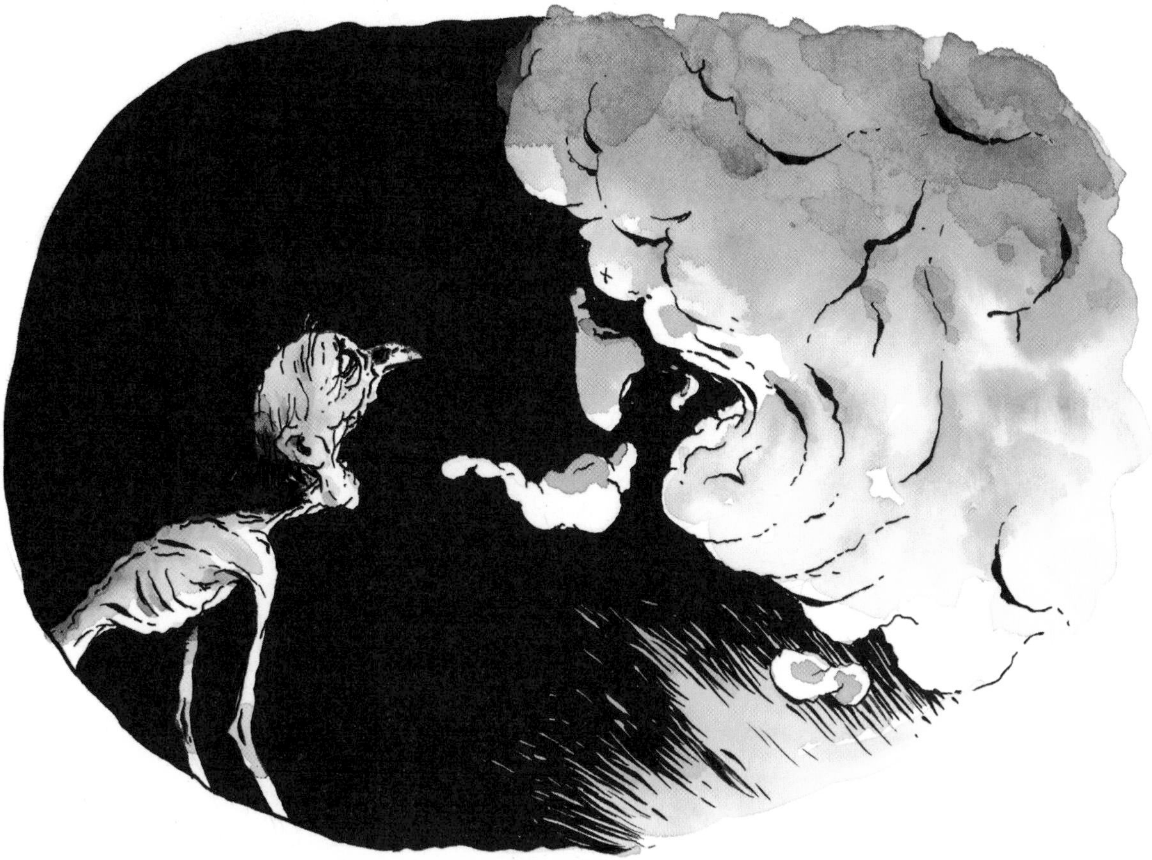

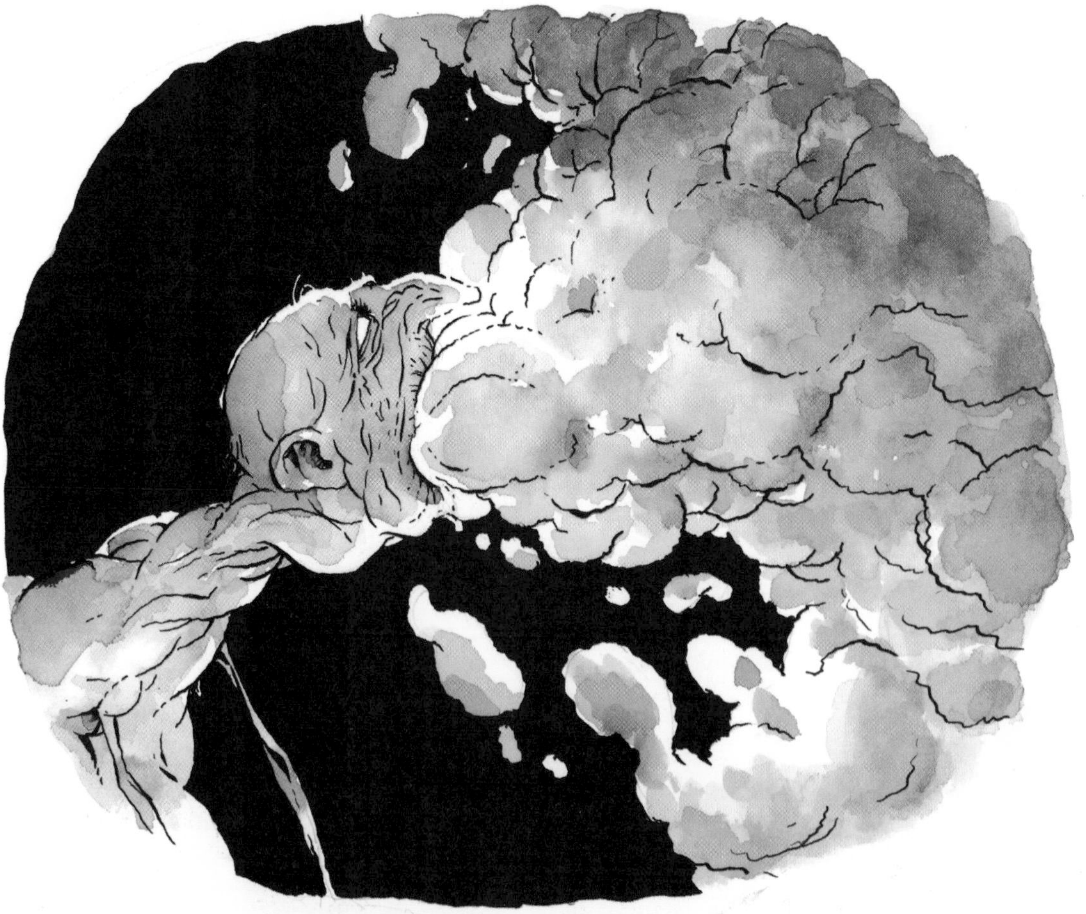

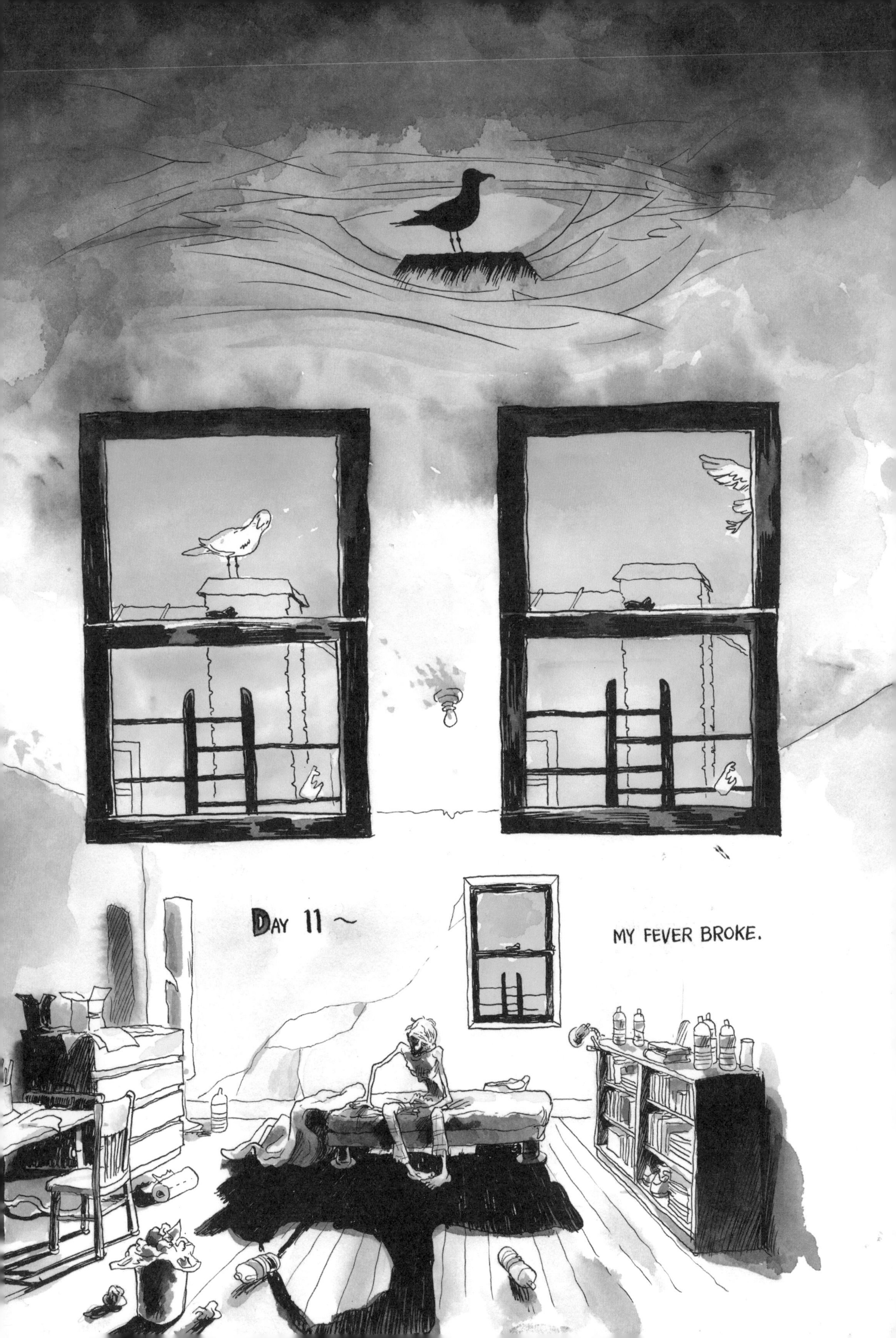
DAY 11 ~
MY FEVER BROKE.

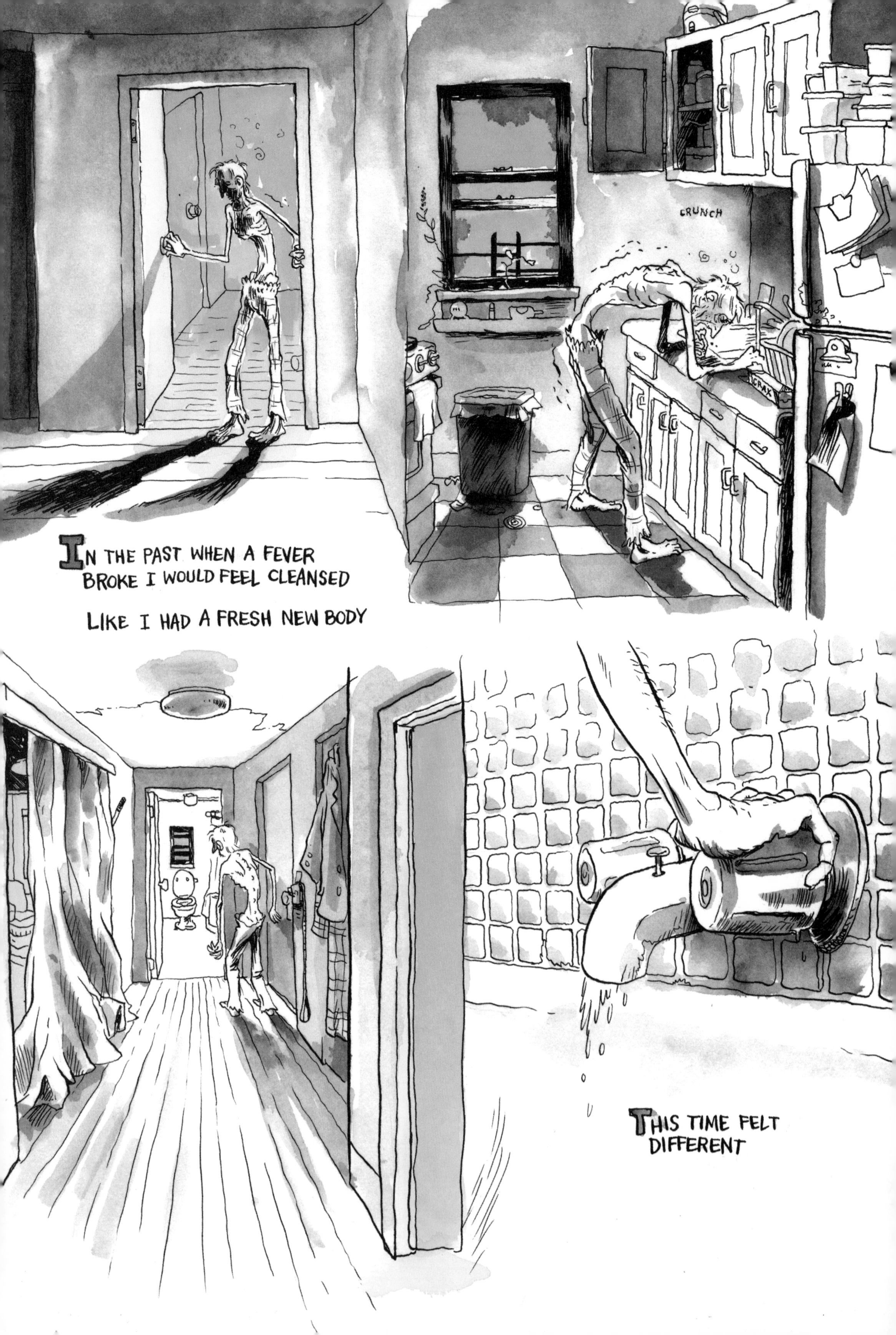
CRUNCH
CRAX
IN THE PAST WHEN A FEVER BROKE I WOULD FEEL CLEANSED
LIKE I HAD A FRESH NEW BODY
THIS TIME FELT DIFFERENT

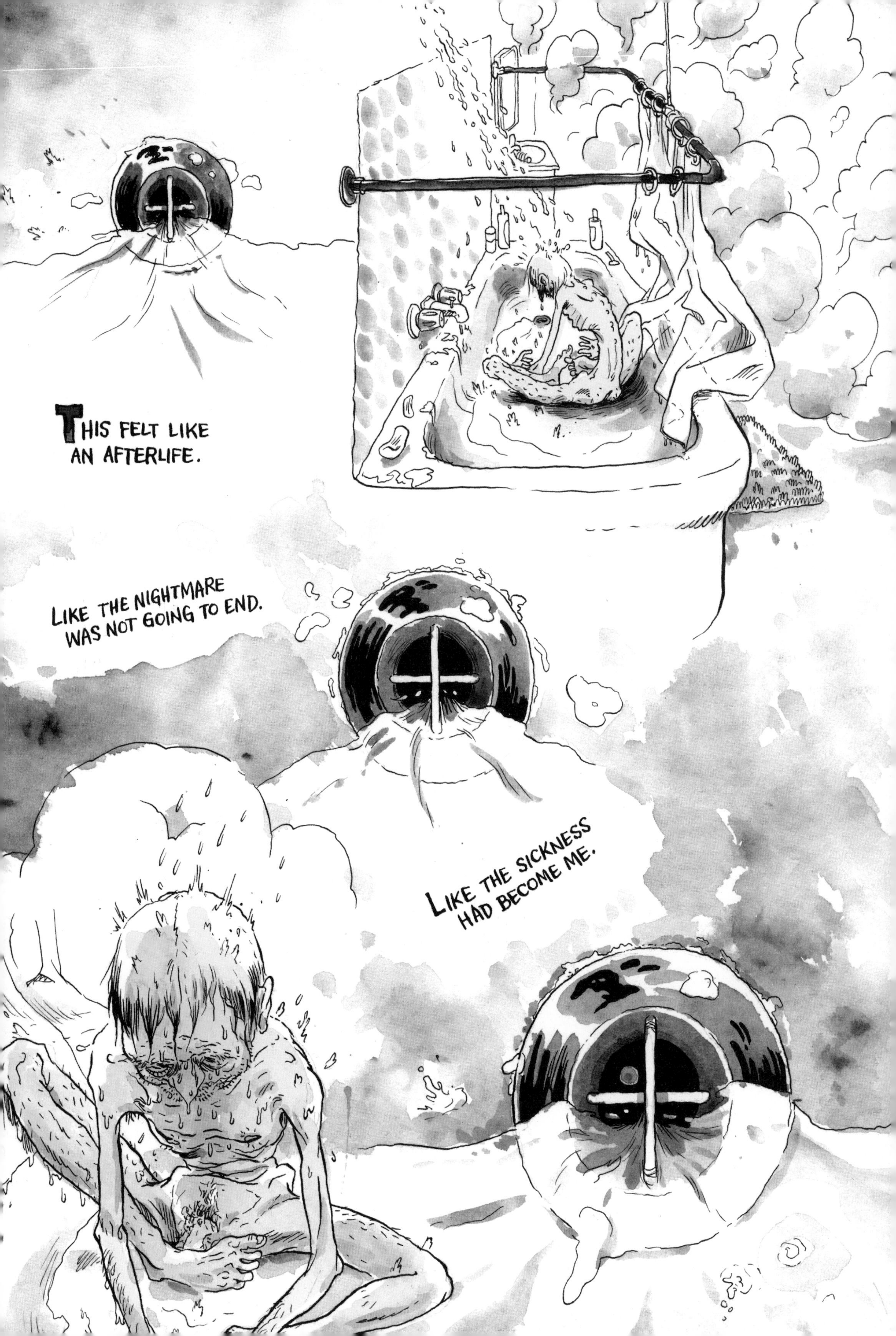
THIS FELT LIKE AN AFTERLIFE.
LIKE THE NIGHTMARE WAS NOT GOING TO END.
LIKE THE SICKNESS HAD BECOME ME.

LOOK AT WHAT PEOPLE LIKE ME
HAVE DONE TO THE WORLD.

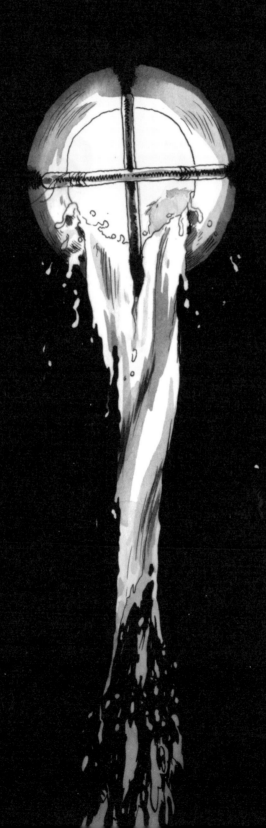

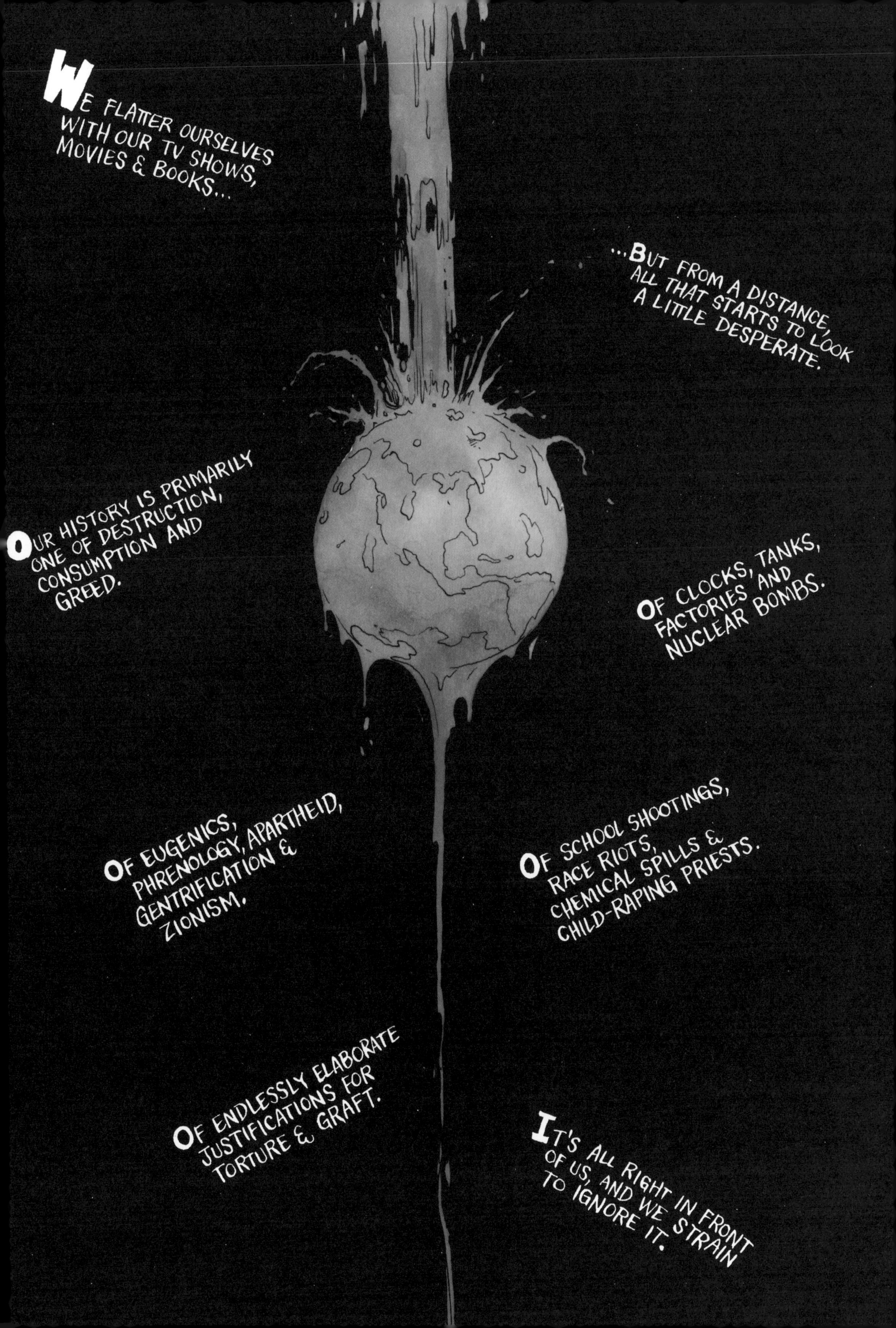
WE FLATTER OURSELVES WITH OUR TV SHOWS, MOVIES & BOOKS...
...BUT FROM A DISTANCE, ALL THAT STARTS TO LOOK A LITTLE DESPERATE.
OUR HISTORY IS PRIMARILY ONE OF DESTRUCTION, CONSUMPTION AND GREED.
OF CLOCKS, TANKS, FACTORIES AND NUCLEAR BOMBS.
OF EUGENICS, PHRENOLOGY, APARTHEID, GENTRIFICATION & ZIONISM.
OF SCHOOL SHOOTINGS, RACE RIOTS, CHEMICAL SPILLS & CHILD-RAPING PRIESTS.
OF ENDLESSLY ELABORATE JUSTIFICATIONS FOR TORTURE & GRAFT.
IT'S ALL RIGHT IN FRONT OF US, AND WE STRAIN TO IGNORE IT.

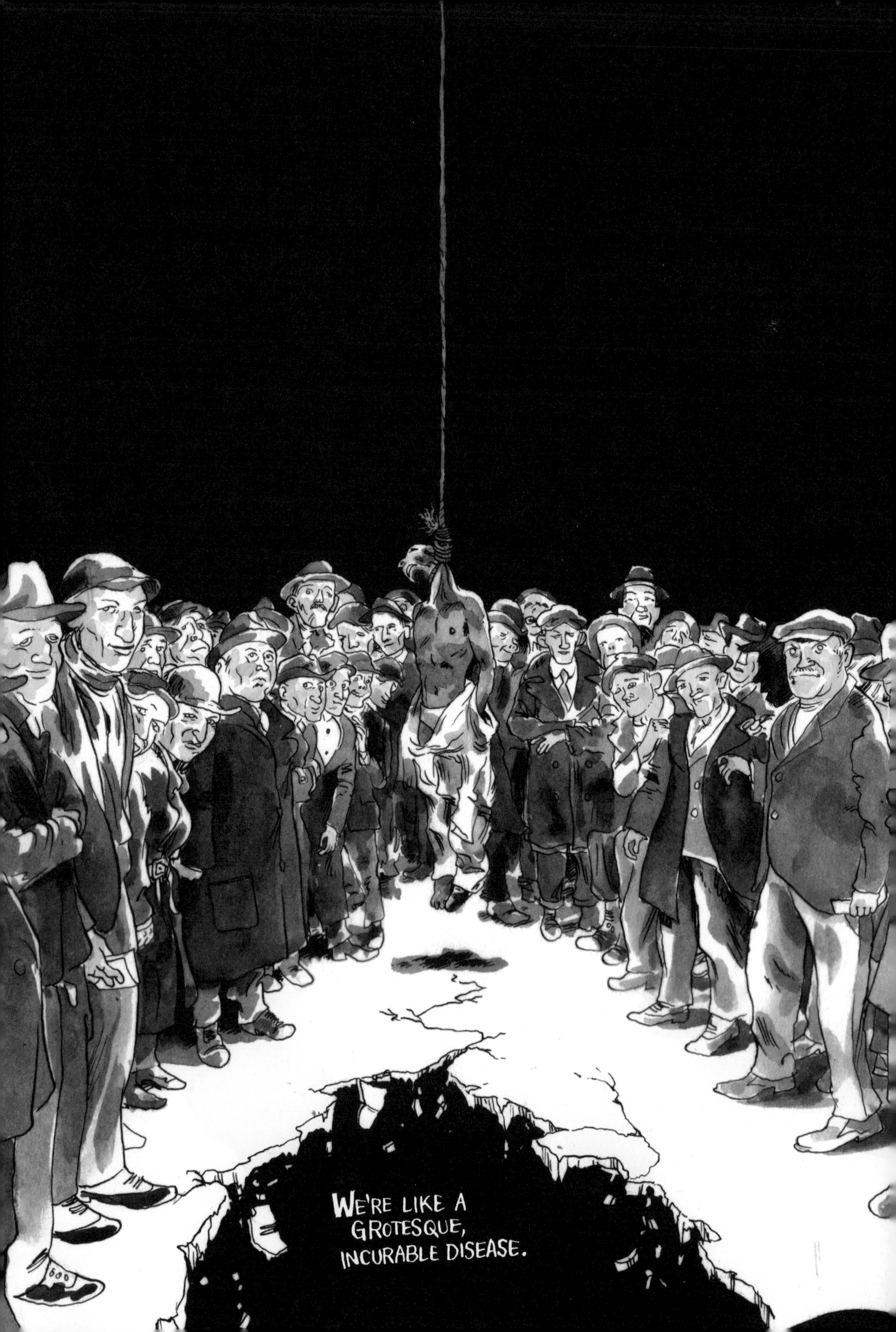
WE'RE LIKE A GROTESQUE, INCURABLE DISEASE.

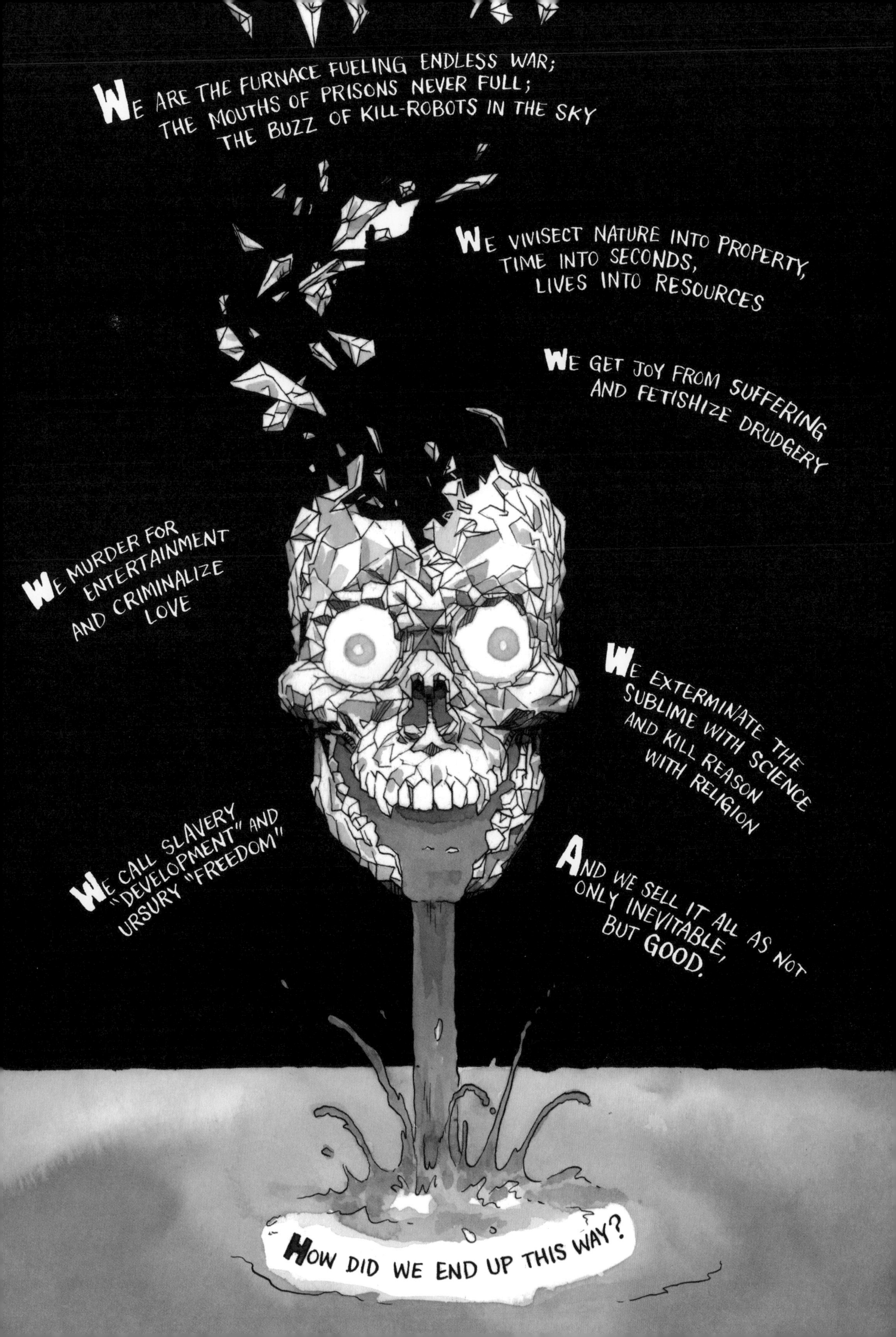
WE ARE THE FURNACE FUELING ENDLESS WAR;
THE MOUTHS OF PRISONS NEVER FULL;
THE BUZZ OF KILL-ROBOTS IN THE SKY
WE VIVISECT NATURE INTO PROPERTY,
TIME INTO SECONDS,
LIVES INTO RESOURCES
WE GET JOY FROM SUFFERING
AND FETISHIZE DRUDGERY
WE MURDER FOR ENTERTAINMENT
AND CRIMINALIZE LOVE
WE EXTERMINATE THE SUBLIME WITH SCIENCE
AND KILL REASON WITH RELIGION
WE CALL SLAVERY "DEVELOPMENT" AND
URSURY "FREEDOM"
AND WE SELL IT ALL AS NOT ONLY INEVITABLE,
BUT GOOD.
HOW DID WE END UP THIS WAY?

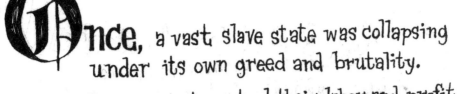

Once, a vast slave state was collapsing under its own greed and brutality.

Desperate to control their labor and profit, the rulers made up a lie that they were gods.

With a little coercion, it worked.

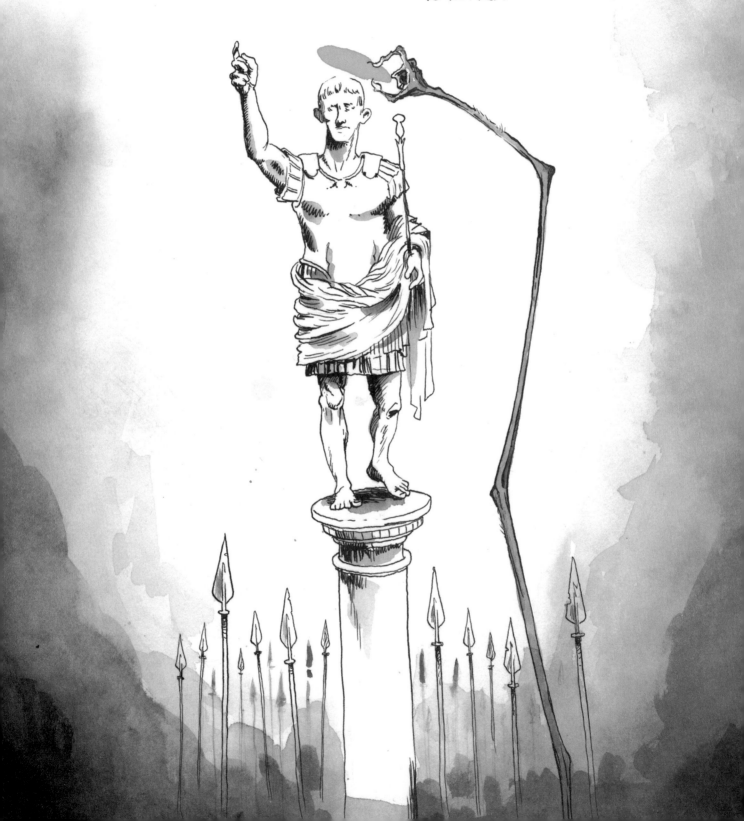

It worked so well that the empire's lower castes had to make their own god-lies in defense.

Soon the empire was full of rival death cults killing each other to see whose lie worked best.

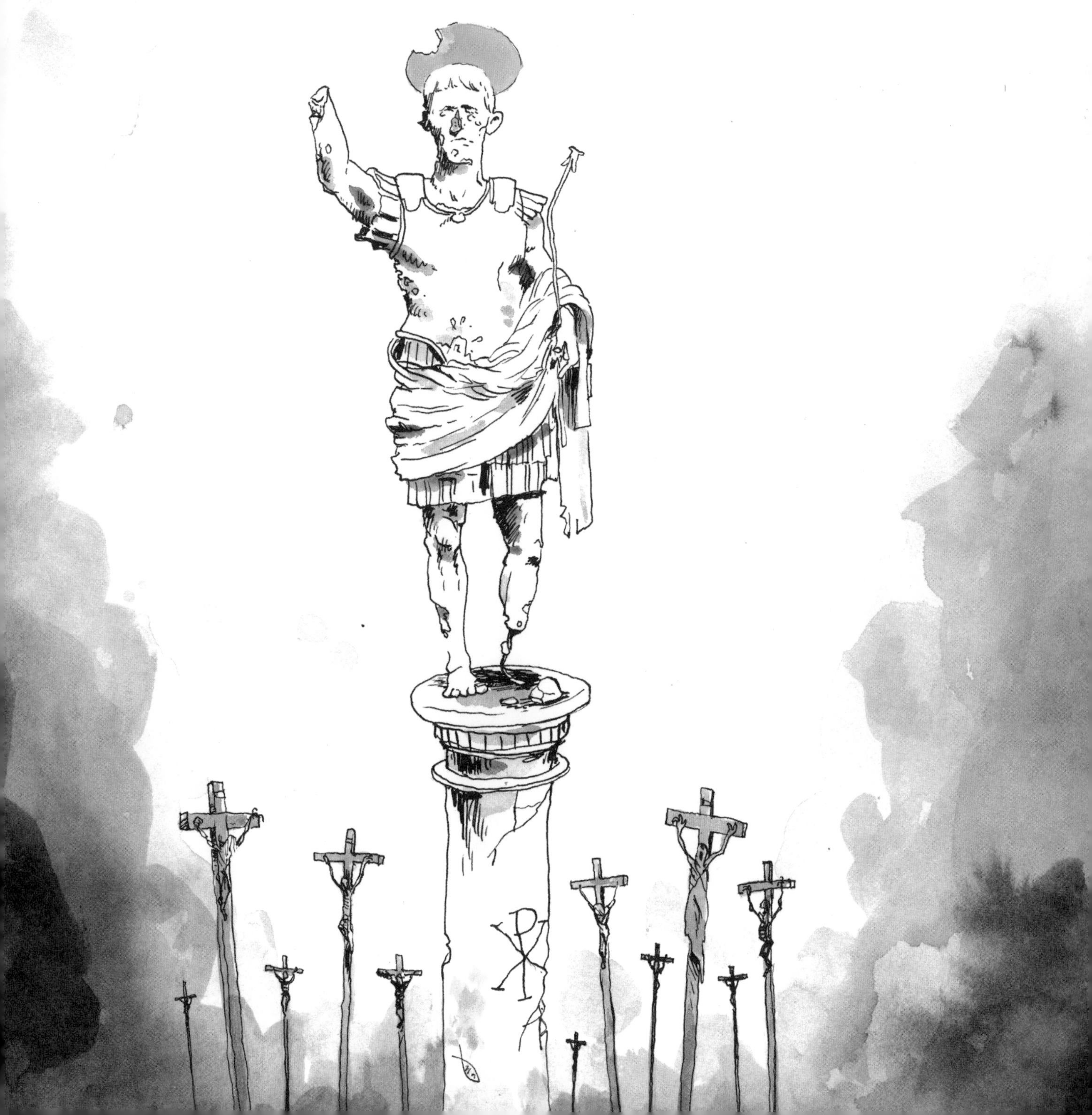

One death cult made up an especially potent lie. Their god wanted to control everything everywhere. He took the shape of a virus and promised infinite power to anyone who let him parasitize and control their body.

This lie worked so well it took over the whole empire.

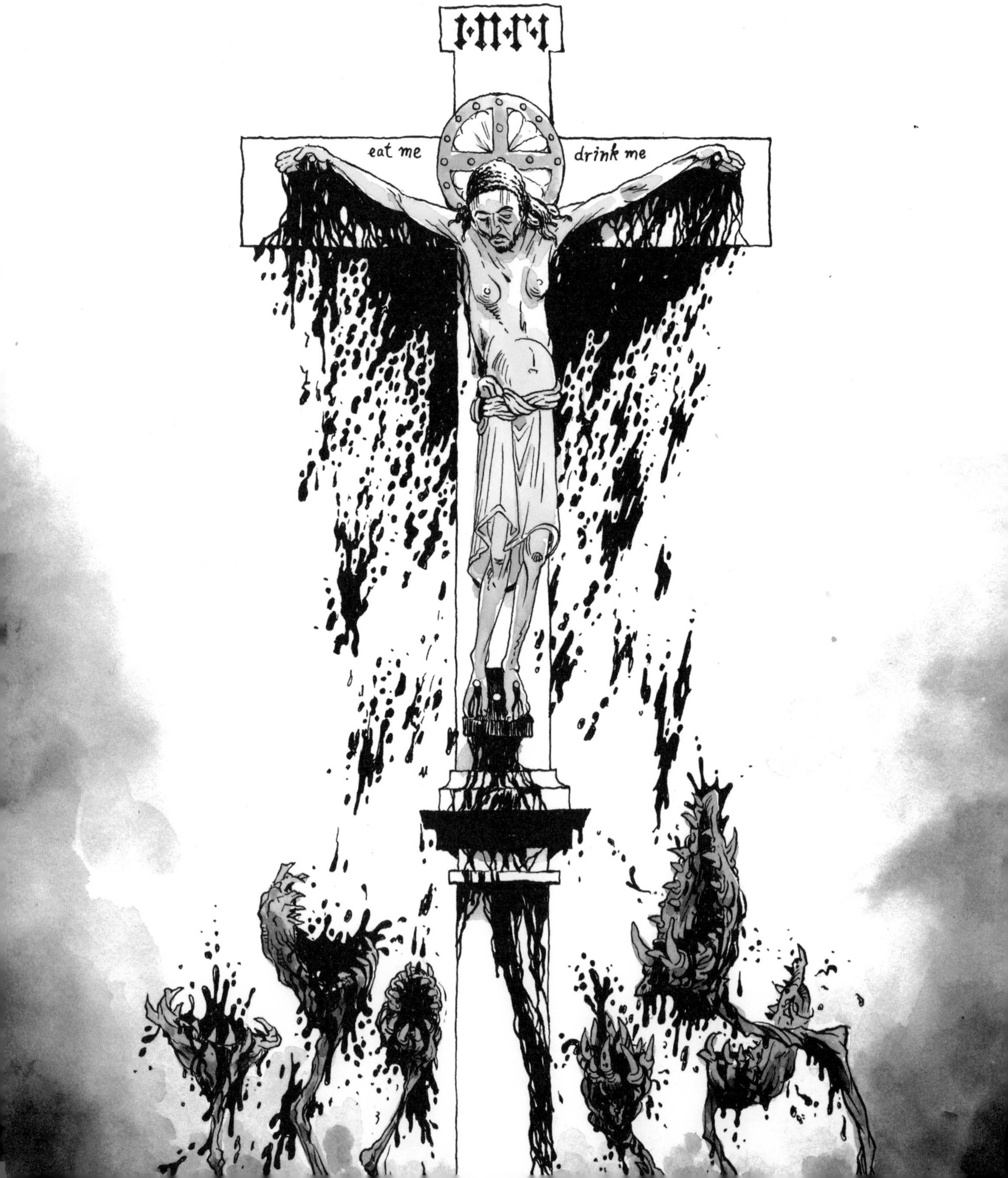
I·N·R·I
eat me
drink me

The virus made life simple, like itself.

As the lie spread across Europe, its power grew and evolved ~ reducing existence to perpetual war.

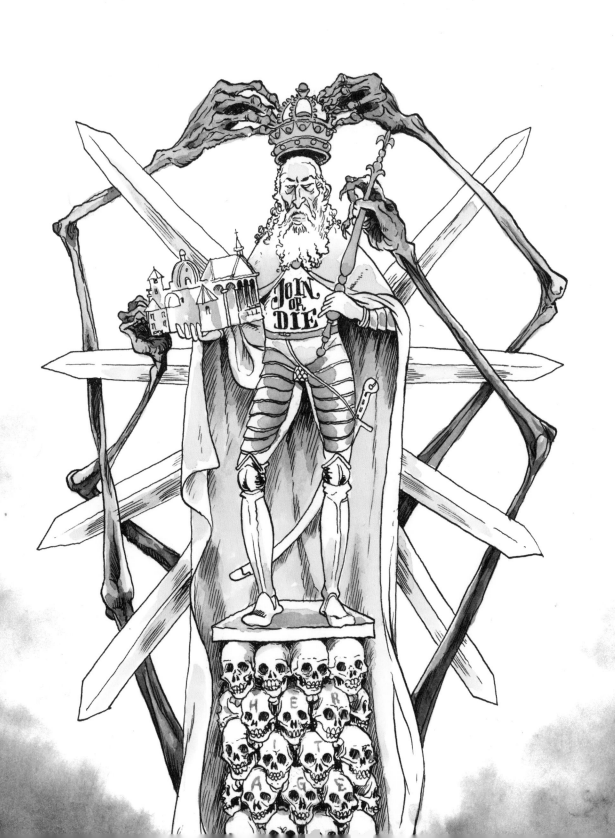

Soon the lie grew so virulent that it infected the whole planet.

The few not destroyed by the virus were taught to sing its simple song, and carry its appetite further into the wilderness.

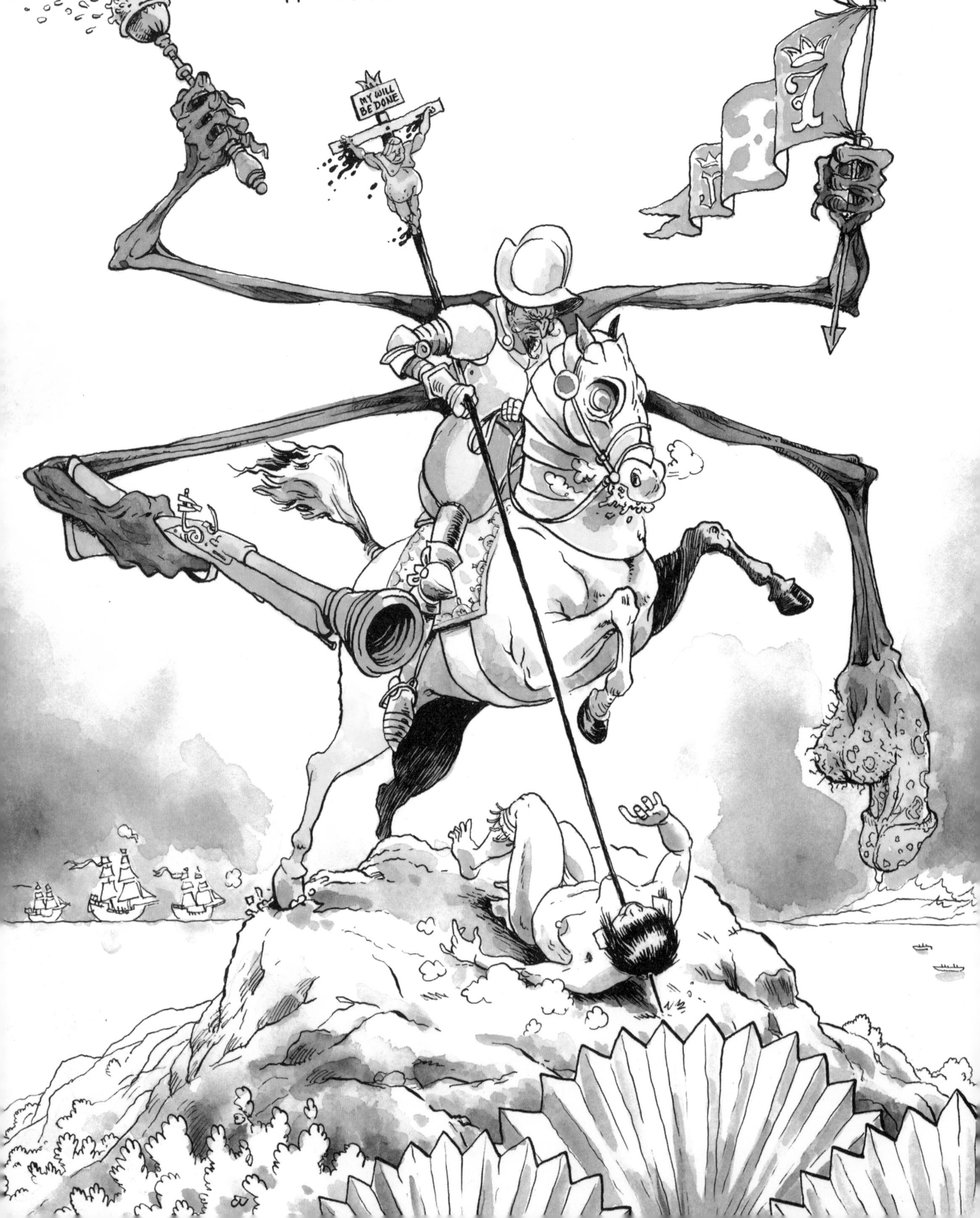
MY WILL BE DONE

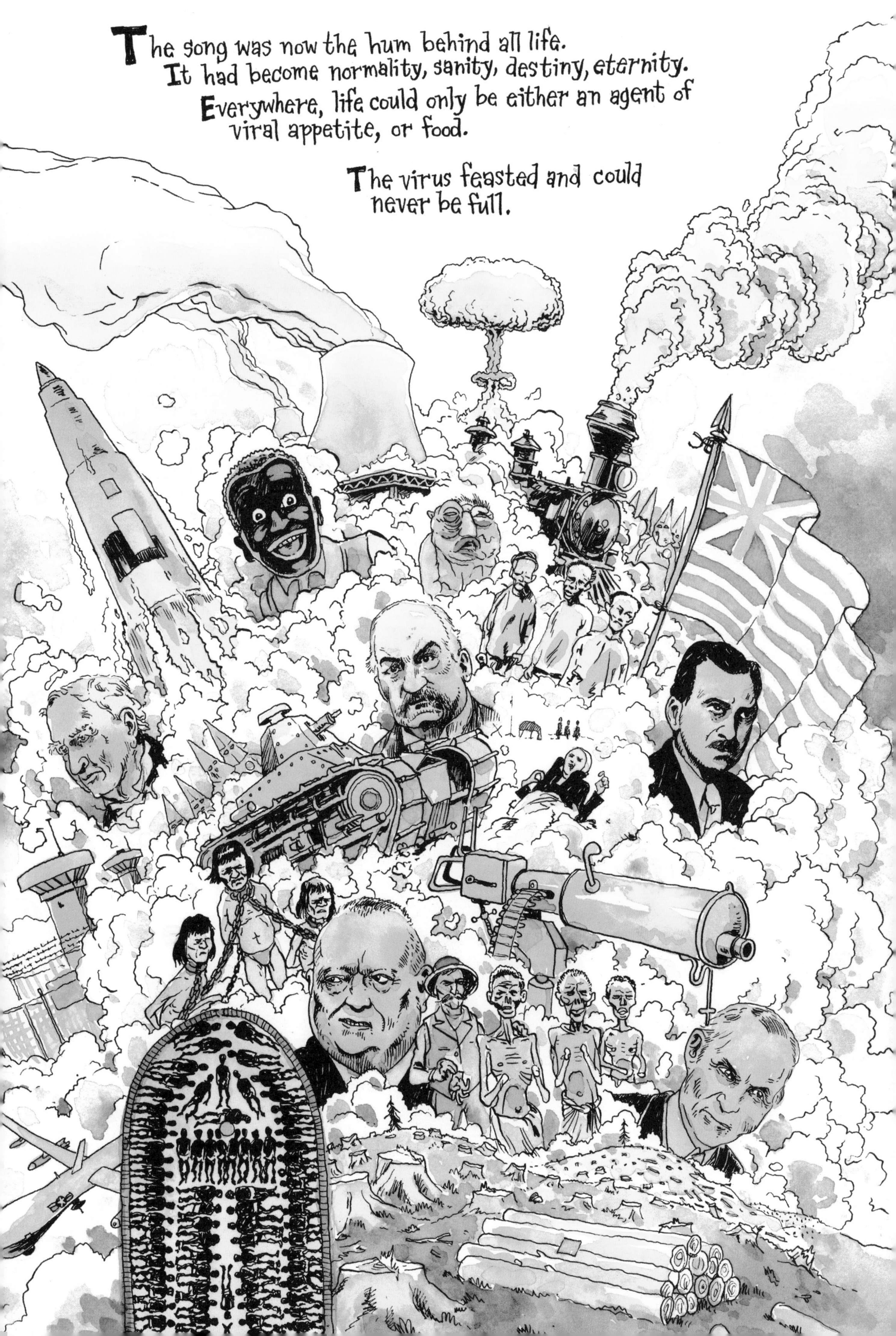
The song was now the hum behind all life.
It had become normality, sanity, destiny, eternity.
Everywhere, life could only be either an agent of viral appetite, or food.
The virus feasted and could never be full.

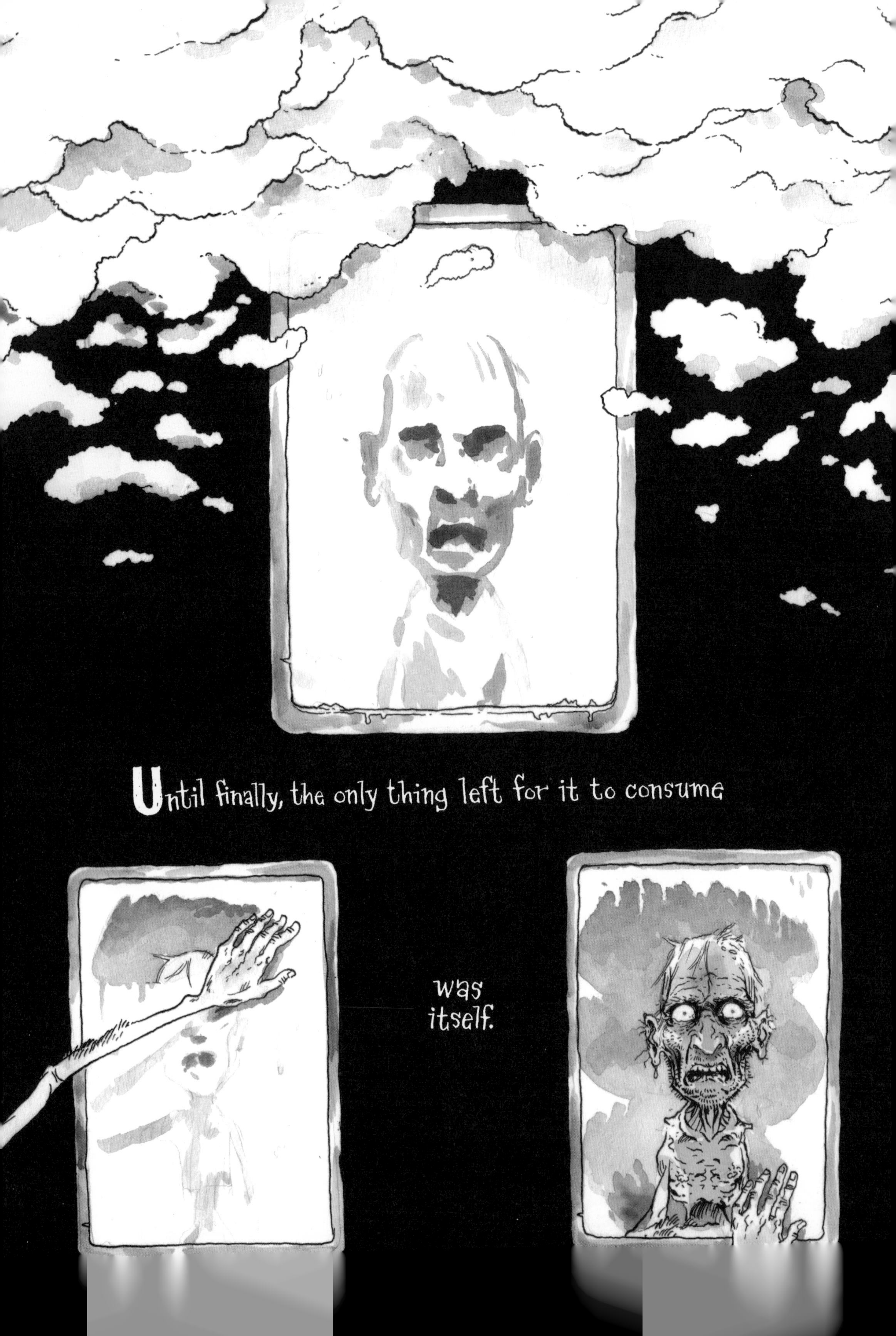
Until finally, the only thing left for it to consume
was
itself.

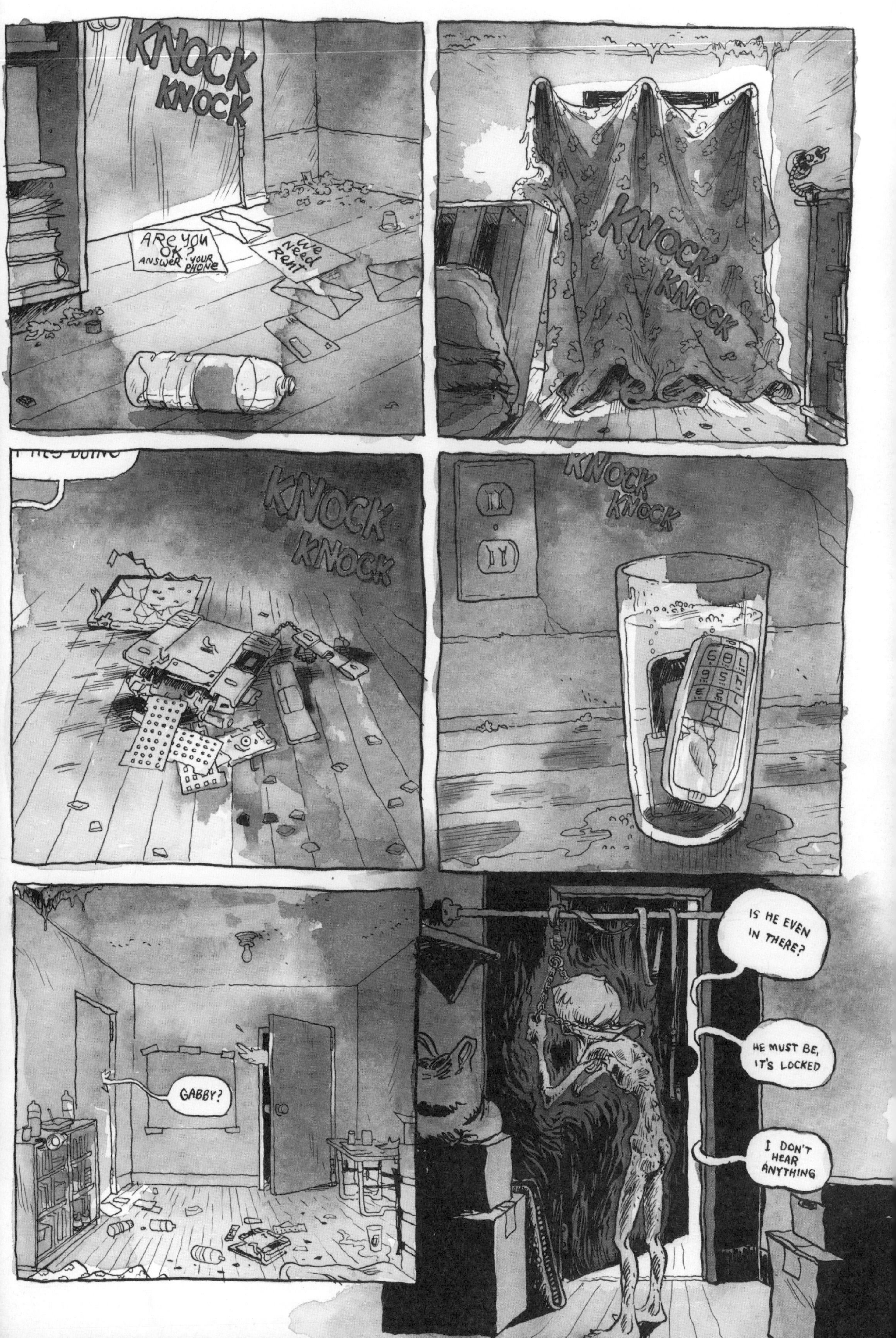
KNOCK KNOCK
ARE YOU OK? ANSWER YOUR PHONE
WE NEED RENT
KNOCK KNOCK
KNOCK KNOCK
KNOCK KNOCK
GABBY?
IS HE EVEN IN THERE?
HE MUST BE, IT'S LOCKED
I DON'T HEAR ANYTHING

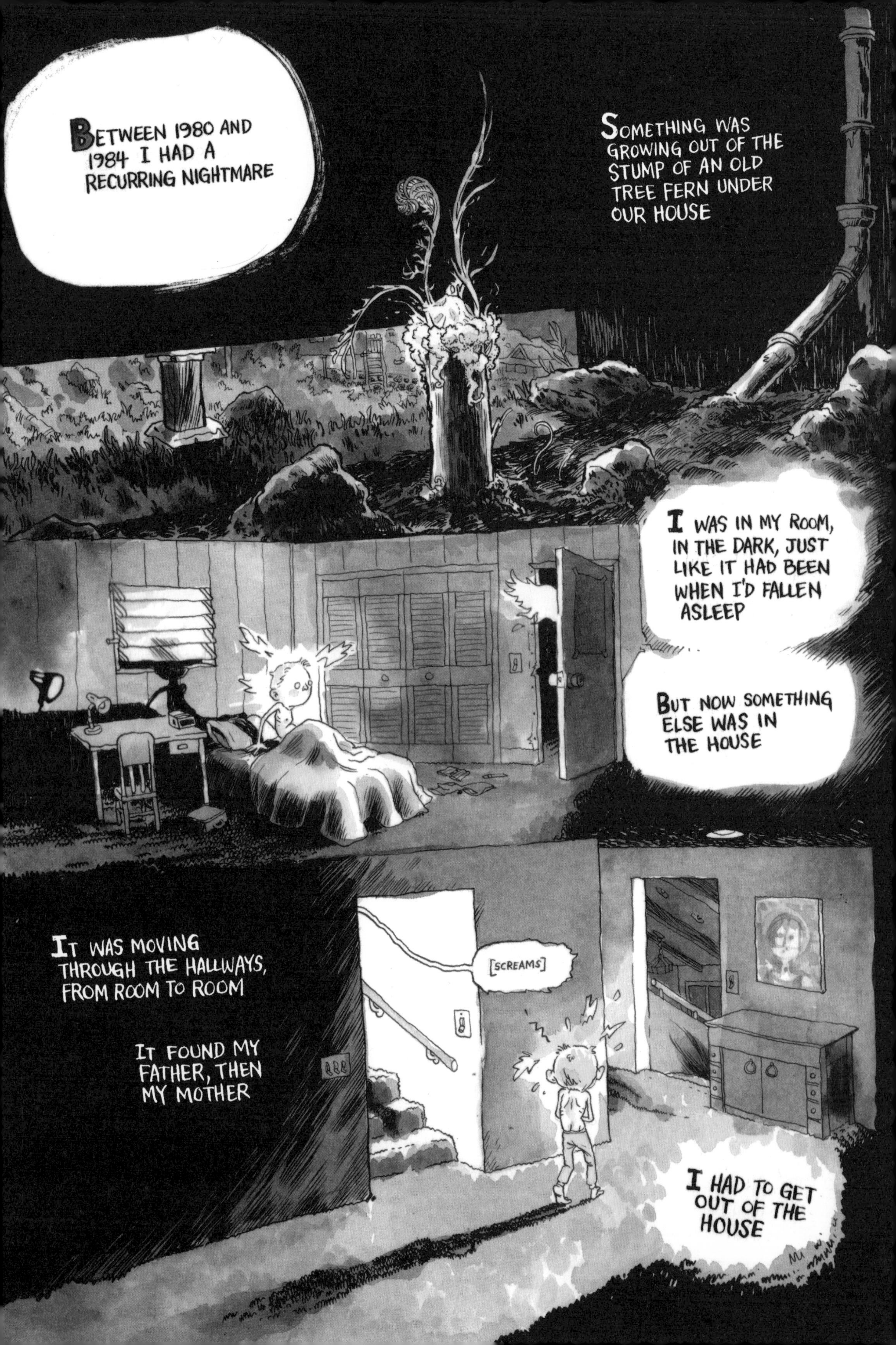
BETWEEN 1980 AND 1984 I HAD A RECURRING NIGHTMARE
SOMETHING WAS GROWING OUT OF THE STUMP OF AN OLD TREE FERN UNDER OUR HOUSE
I WAS IN MY ROOM, IN THE DARK, JUST LIKE IT HAD BEEN WHEN I'D FALLEN ASLEEP
BUT NOW SOMETHING ELSE WAS IN THE HOUSE
IT WAS MOVING THROUGH THE HALLWAYS, FROM ROOM TO ROOM
[SCREAMS]
IT FOUND MY FATHER, THEN MY MOTHER
I HAD TO GET OUT OF THE HOUSE

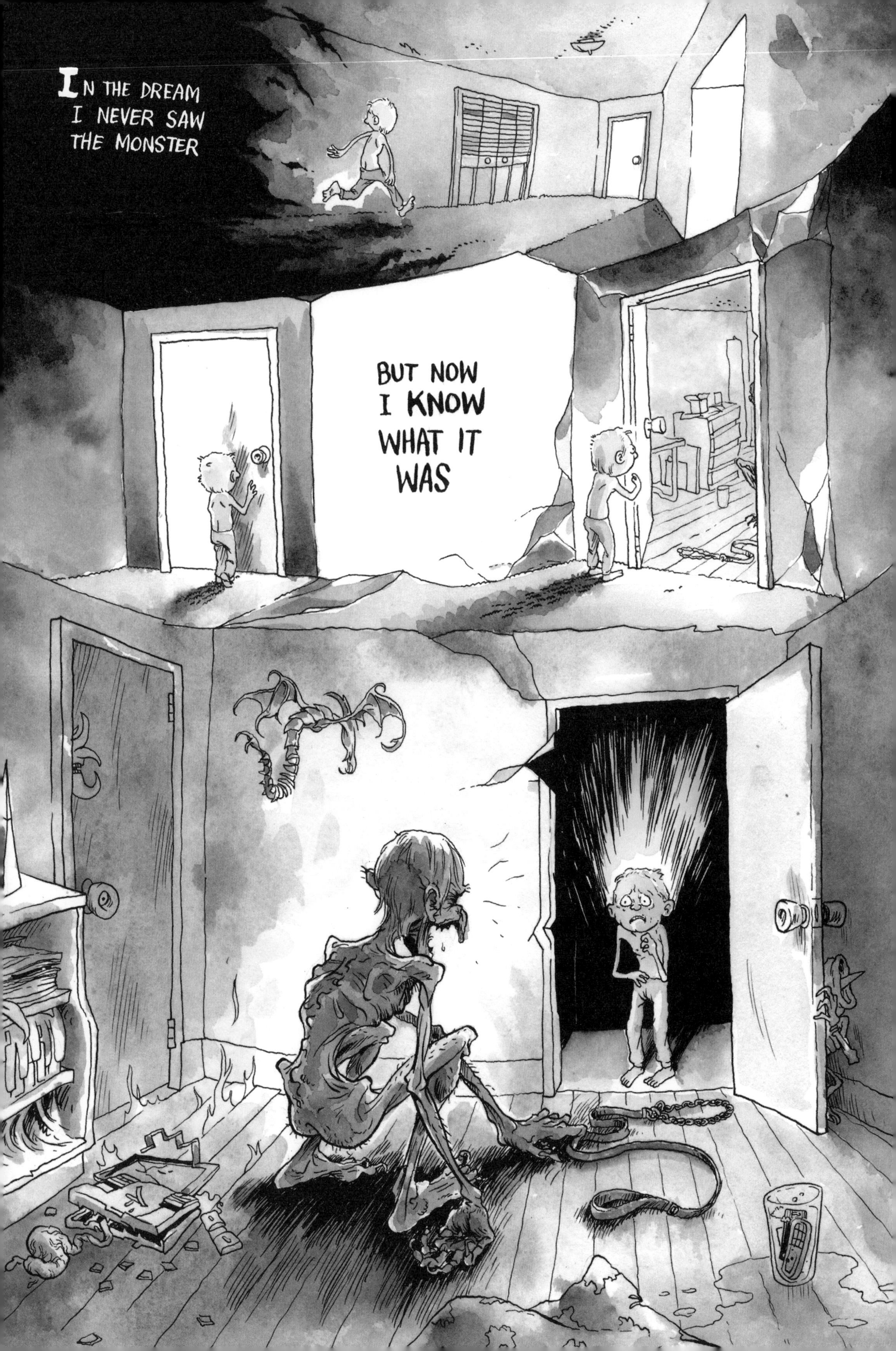
IN THE DREAM
I NEVER SAW
THE MONSTER
BUT NOW
I KNOW
WHAT IT
WAS

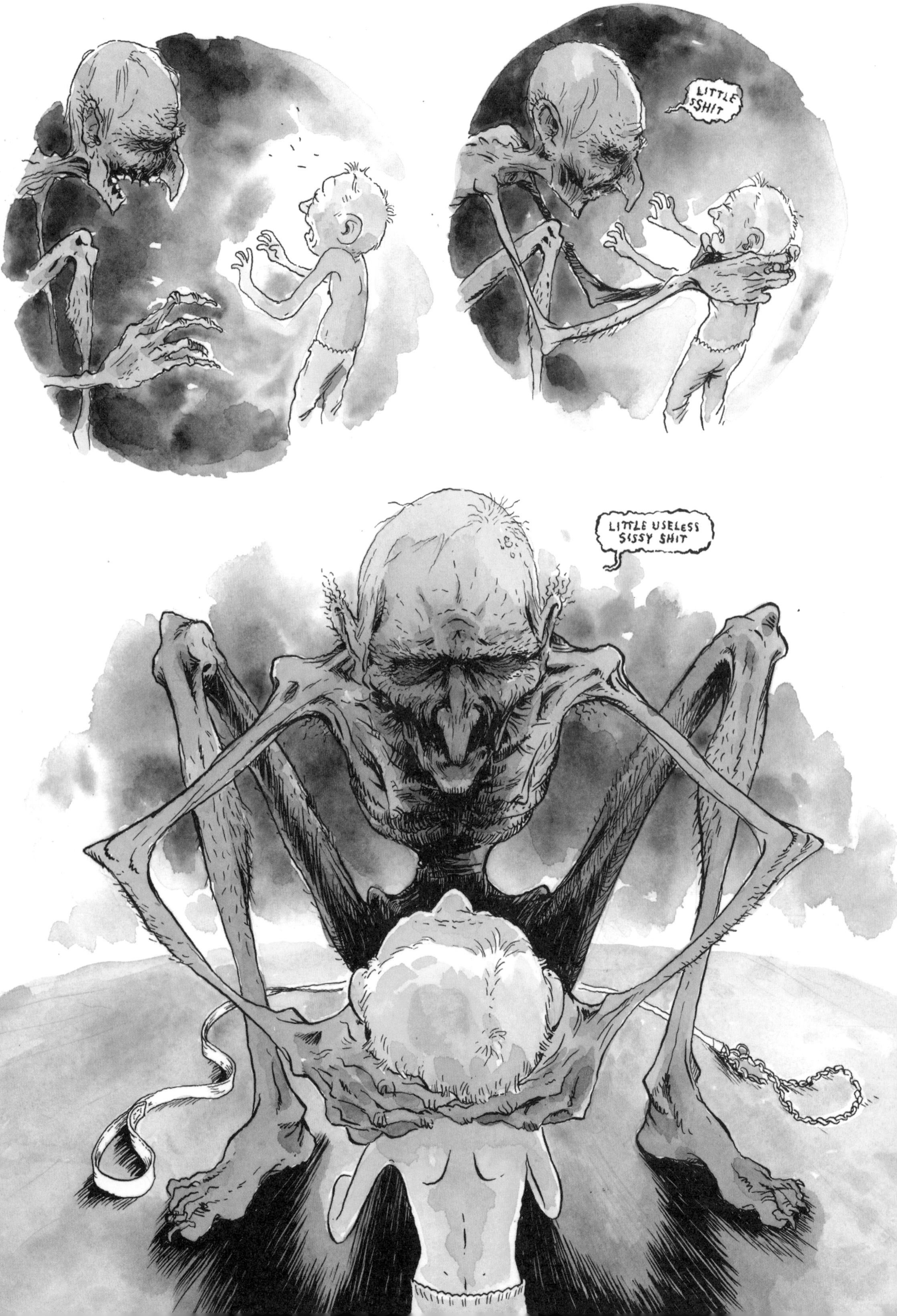
LITTLE SSHIT
LITTLE USELESS SISSY SHIT

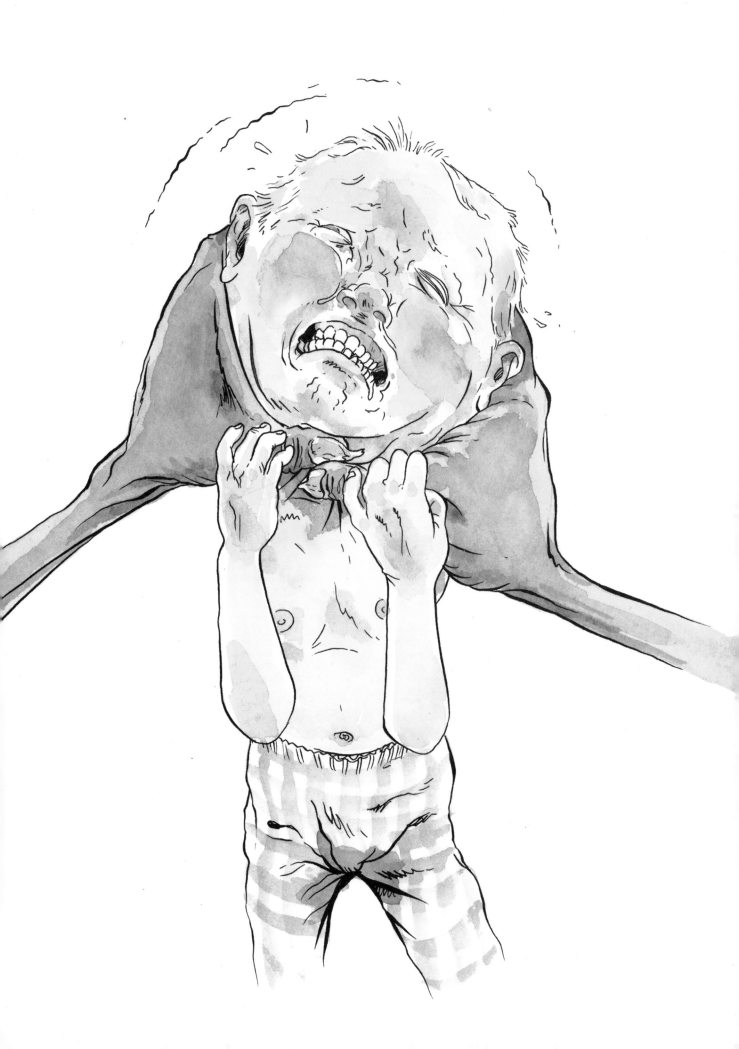

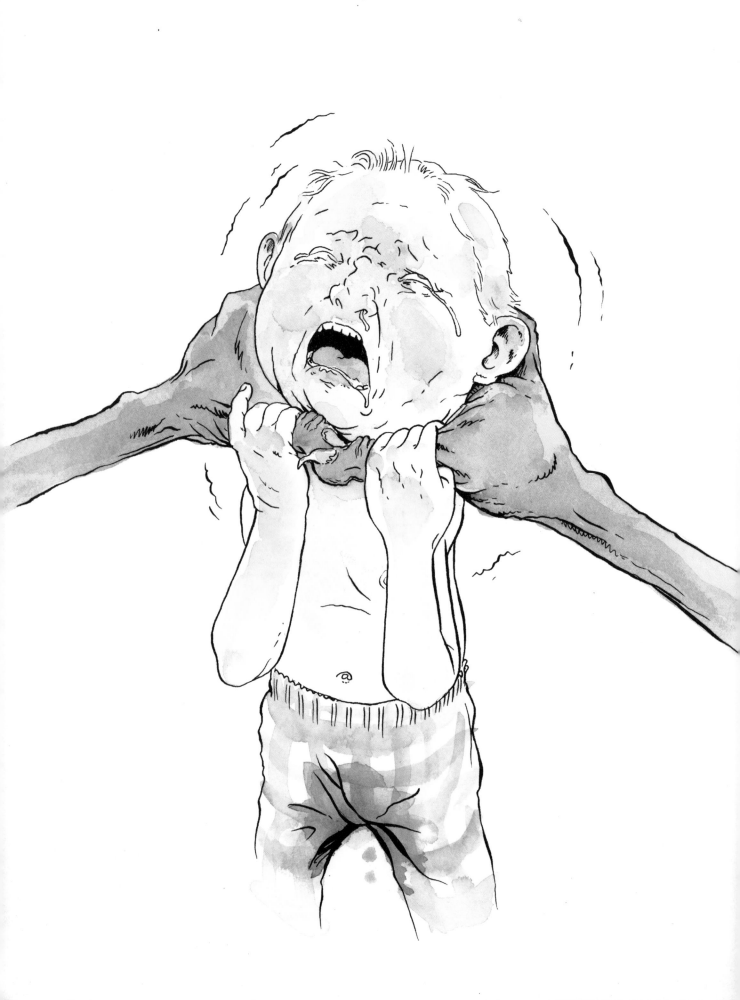

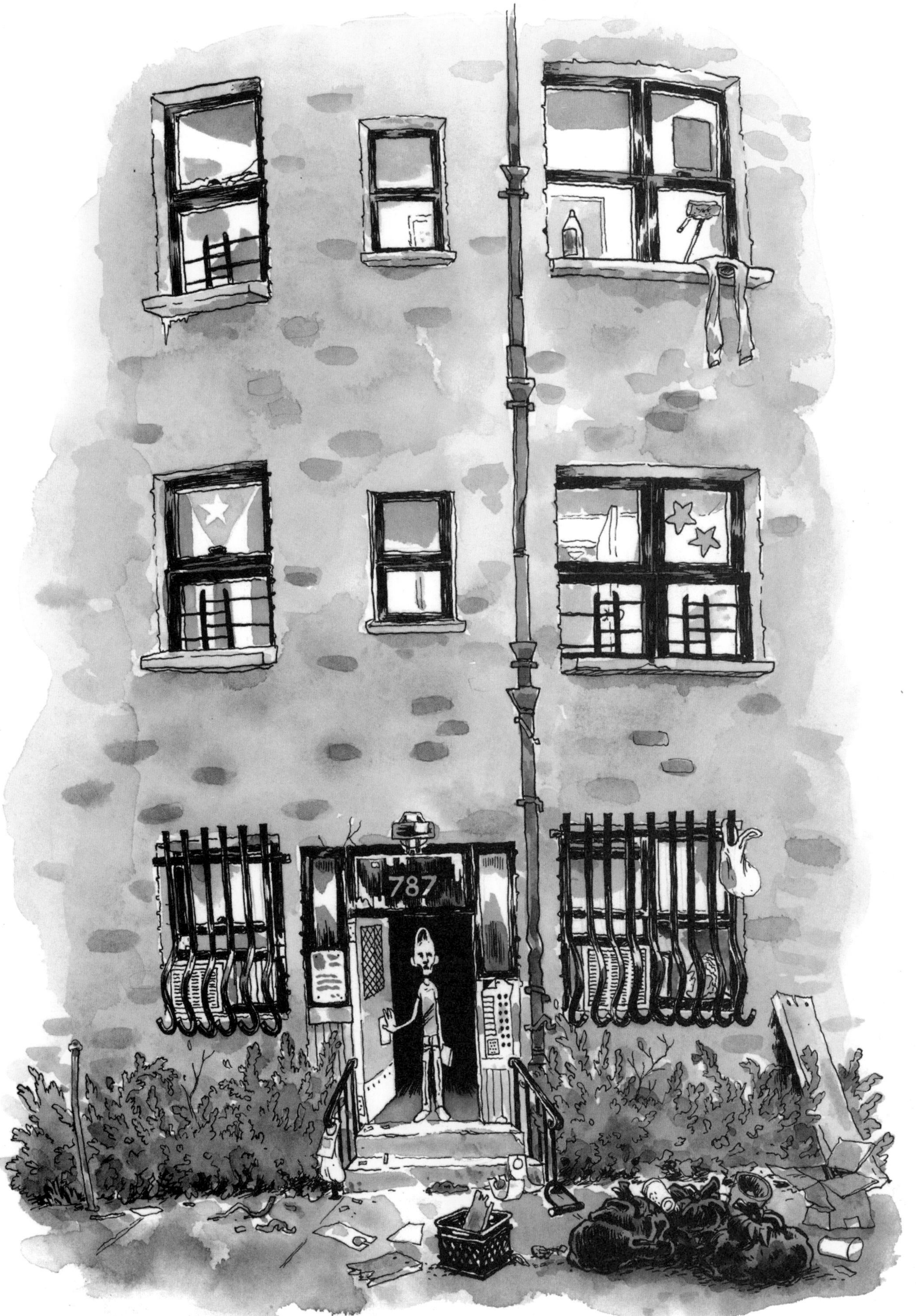
787

DAY 15

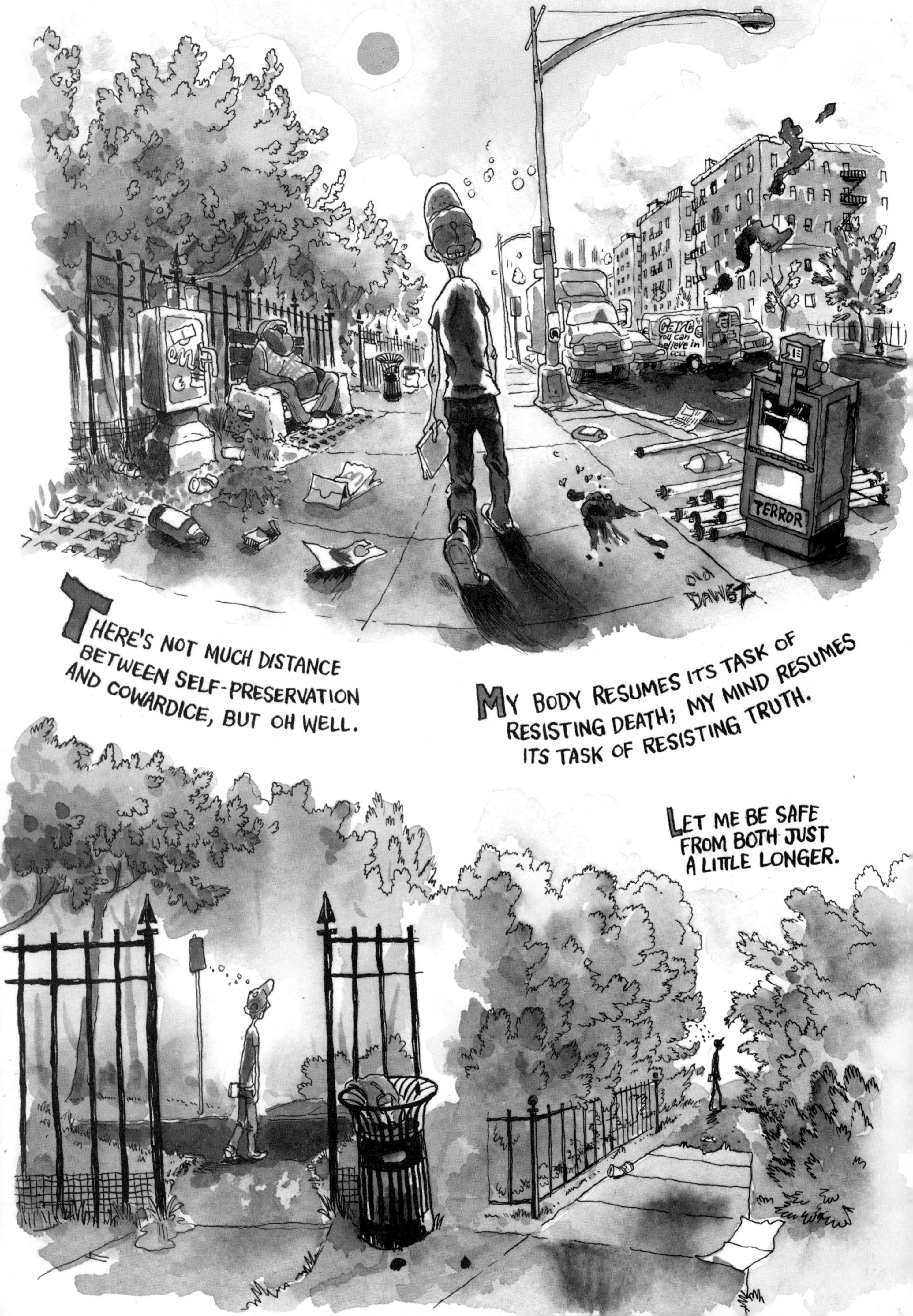
TERROR
THERE'S NOT MUCH DISTANCE BETWEEN SELF-PRESERVATION AND COWARDICE, BUT OH WELL.
MY BODY RESUMES ITS TASK OF RESISTING DEATH; MY MIND RESUMES ITS TASK OF RESISTING TRUTH.
LET ME BE SAFE FROM BOTH JUST A LITTLE LONGER.

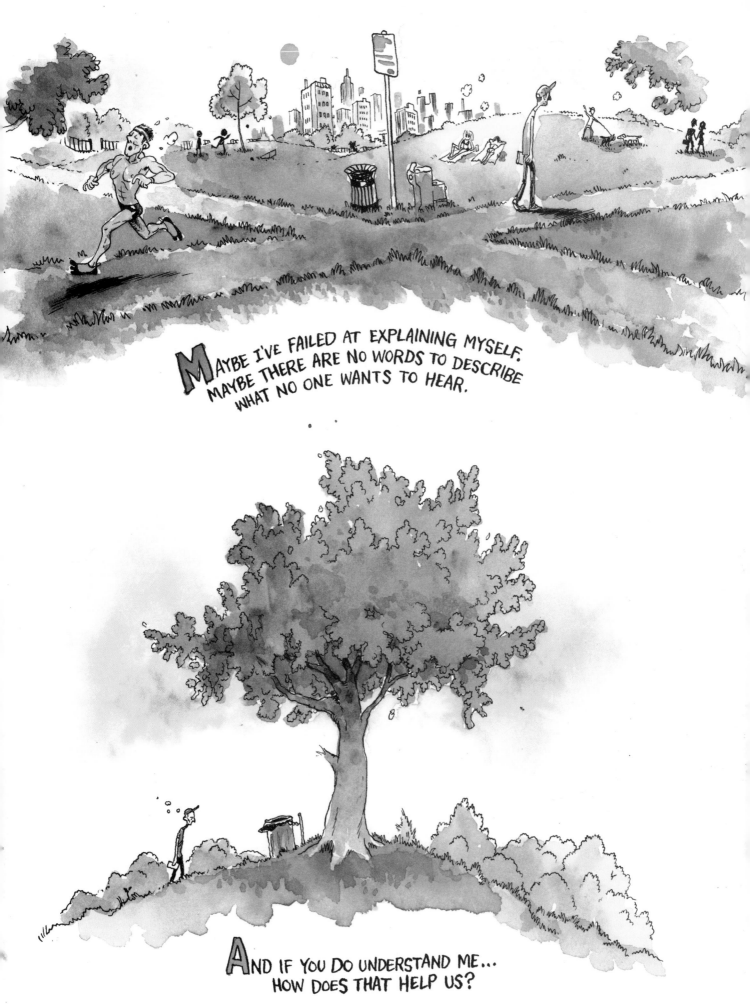

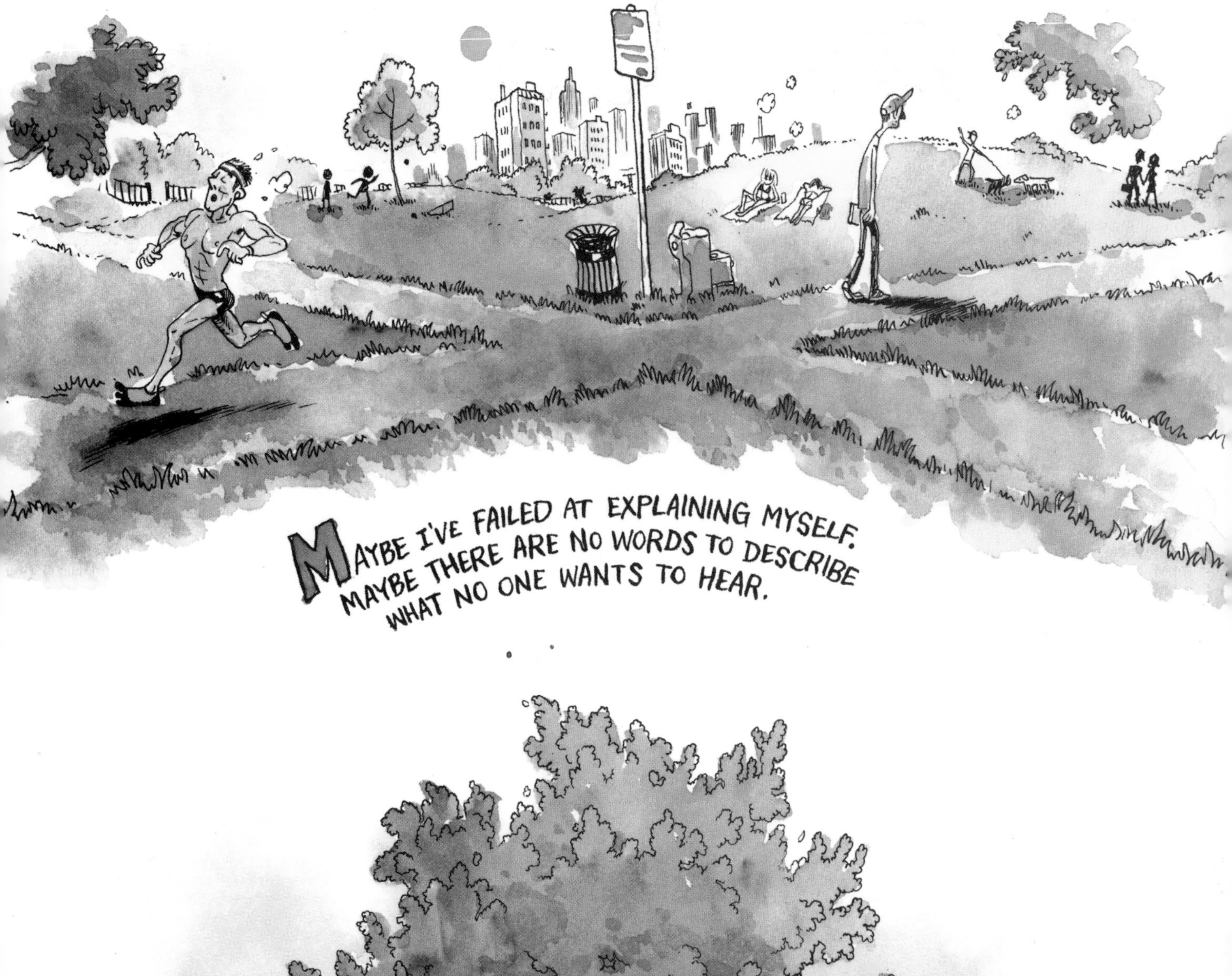
MAYBE I'VE FAILED AT EXPLAINING MYSELF. MAYBE THERE ARE NO WORDS TO DESCRIBE WHAT NO ONE WANTS TO HEAR.
AND IF YOU DO UNDERSTAND ME... HOW DOES THAT HELP US?

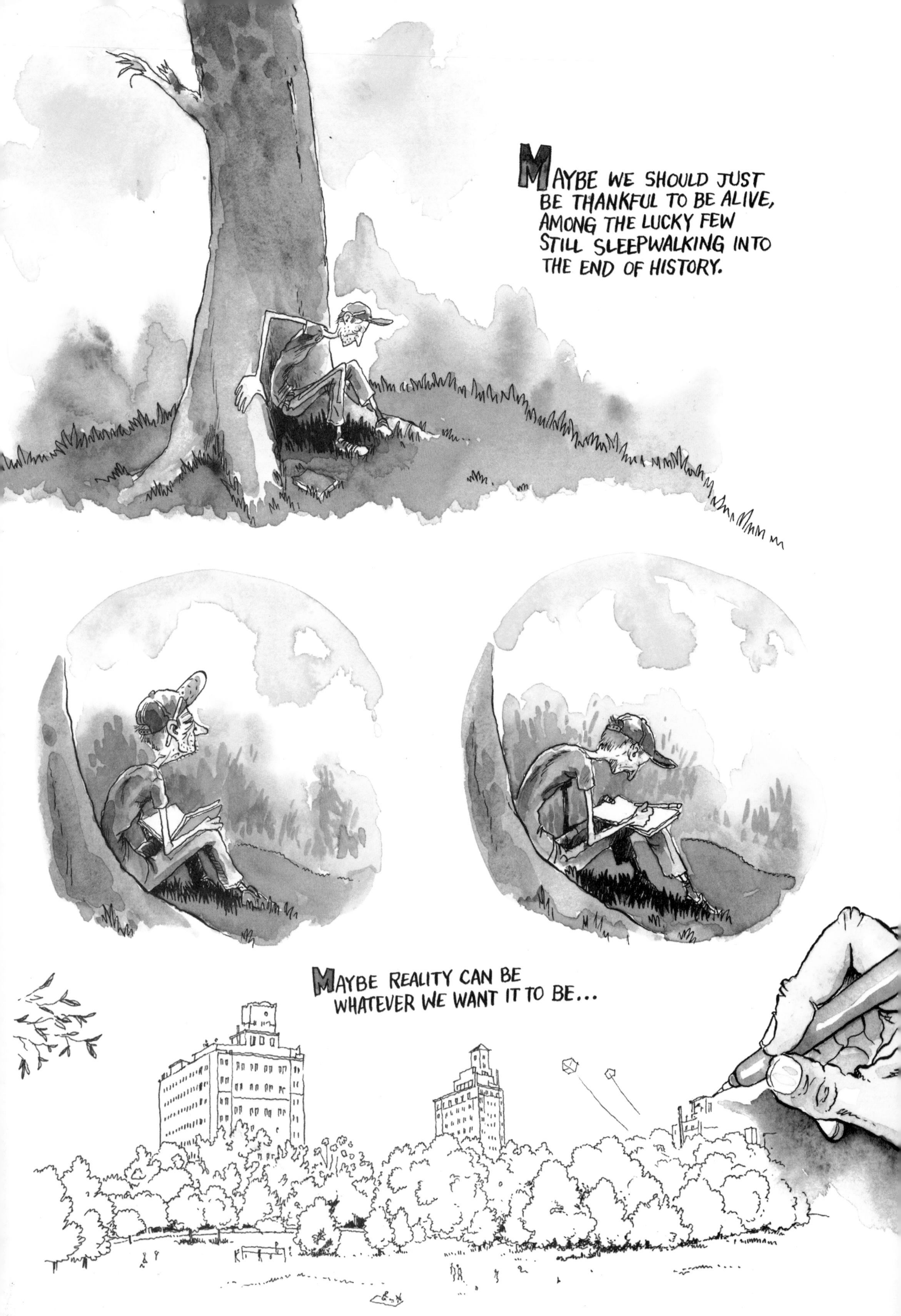
MAYBE WE SHOULD JUST BE THANKFUL TO BE ALIVE, AMONG THE LUCKY FEW STILL SLEEPWALKING INTO THE END OF HISTORY.
MAYBE REALITY CAN BE WHATEVER WE WANT IT TO BE...

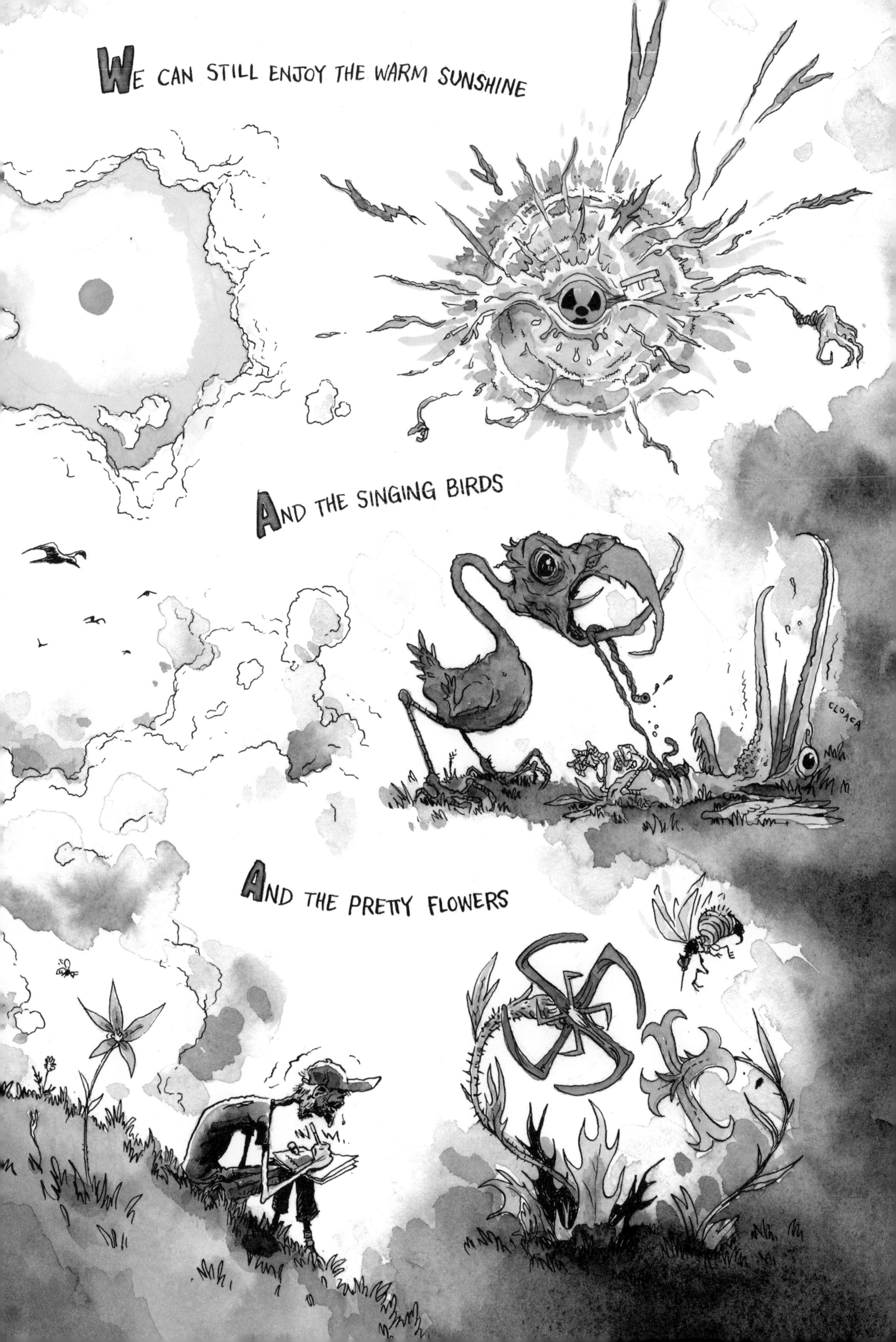
We can still enjoy the warm sunshine
And the singing birds
CLOACA
And the pretty flowers

AND THE PLUG OF HUMAN SKIN AND HAIR I FOUND HIDING IN THE GRASS

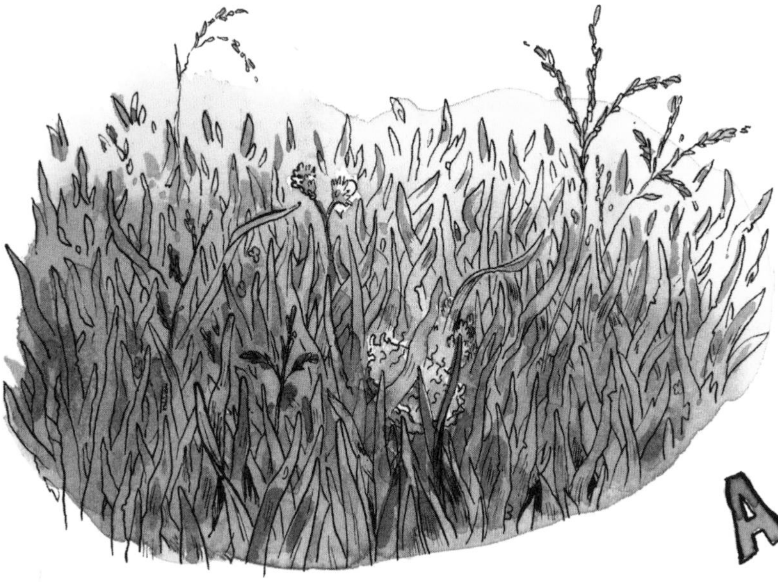

AND ALL THE BEAUTIFUL PEOPLE ENJOYING THIS BEAUTIFUL WORLD

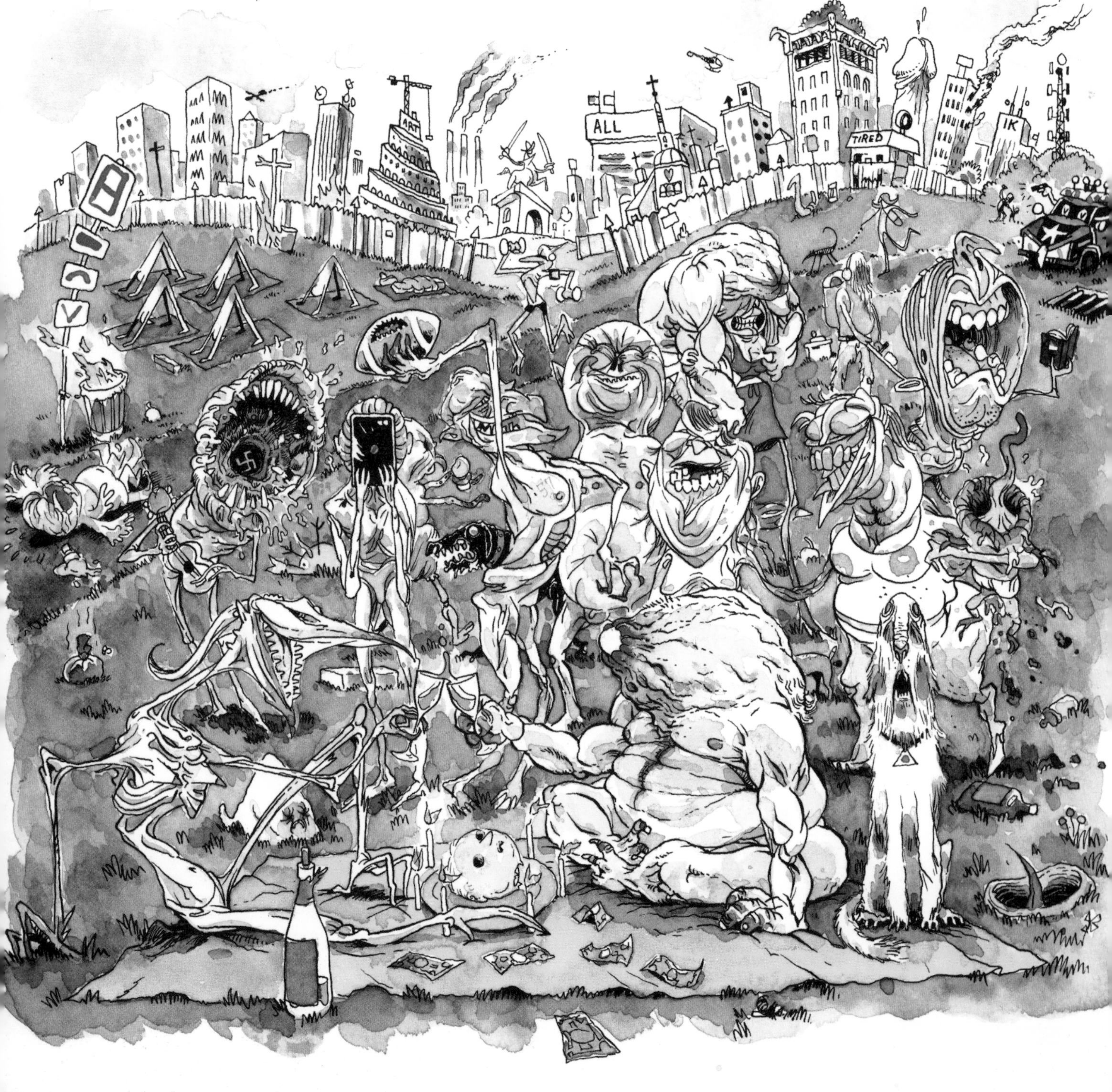
ALL
ART
TIRED

AND IF THIS IS THE LIFE WE'VE MADE FOR OURSELVES

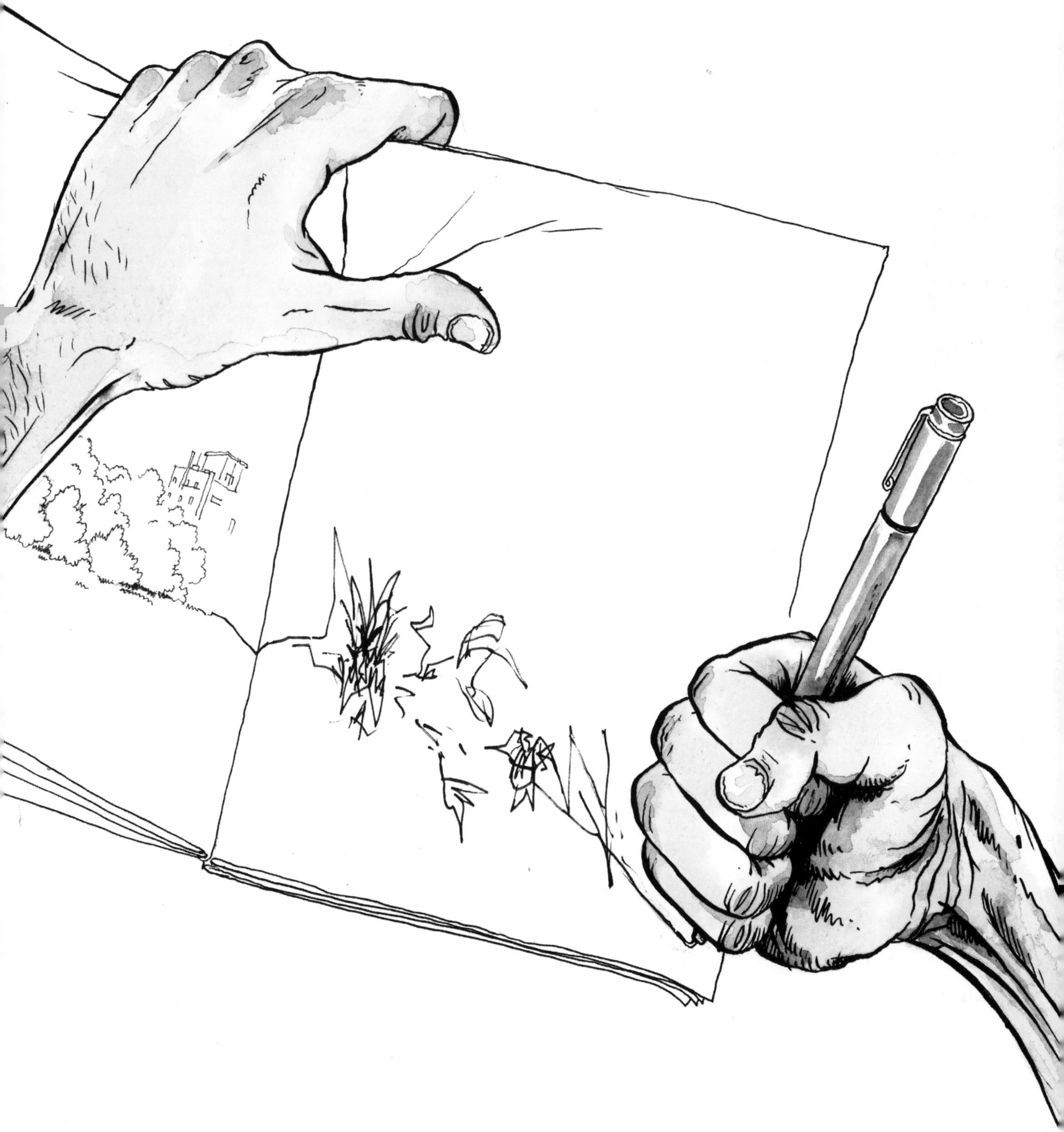

THEN WHAT A FITTING PUNISHMENT TO LIVE IT.

IT'S ALL PRETTY WONDERFUL, REALLY.

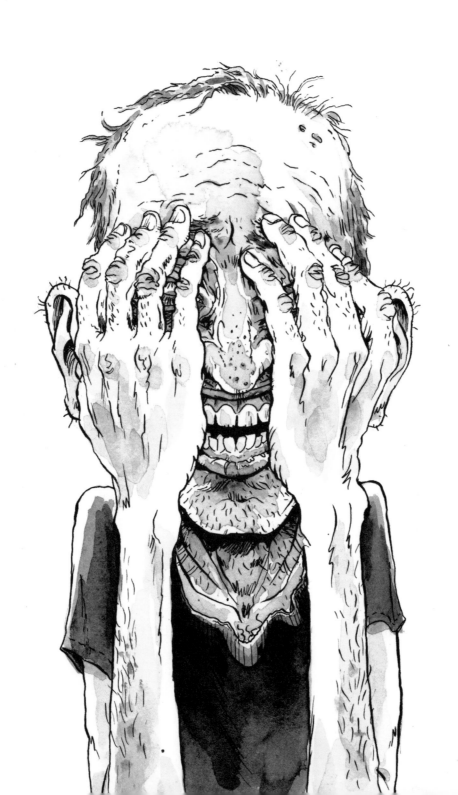

I'm sorry

P.L.
Erin L.
Gordon A.
Miyoko N.
The Kukea family
The man who picked me
   up in downtown
   Phoenix in 1991
The woman stranded with
   me in the Greyhound
   station in Grand
   Junction, CO in 1999
The Sendrow family
Kim H.
Shawn L.
The Sugimoto family
Hiroshi T.
Claire G.
Mike W.
Cade R.
Dayle-Anne L.
Sandra K.
Gabe the punk kid I
   ditched in 1991
Sheung-Shar
Lisa E.
Pat K.
Eliza S.
Daniel R.
Christina Sc.
R.C.
Caitlin M.
Raven C.
Cass W.
Katelyn J.
The Japanese
   exchange student
   in 1979
Stephen S.
Pat M.
The Sue family
The employees of the
   video store in the
   strip mall at King &
   Hauoli in 1982

Kaz S.
Otto
Keith F.
Eugene W.
Harry T.
Chandler & Vanessa
Sacha K.
Heather Q.
Gabrielle B.
Katie B.
Barry M.
Leon A.
Max deR.
Matthias R.
Erica J.
Dane M.
Janet B.
Doug Upp
Stu D.
Sick of the Abuse
Cheyenne N.
Mark Miraflor
Chris W.
Mark Tagal
Galen K.
Jose E.
Liz M.
E.B. & S.B.
Marcelyn S.
Hannah in Crown
   Heights in 2011
John T.
Sam F.
Joanne Yuen
Julie D.
Steve D.
Shannon McN.
Jen C.
Phil
Karen LeB.
The skinny girl from New
   York I dated briefly
   in 1997 then ignored

Lauren D.
Colin H.
Cathy S.
Dawn F.
Rhoda
The employees of
   Matteo's in 1994
Doc B.
J.D. H.
The Yuen family
Patrice at Emilio's
Michelle F.
Mark D.
Marla T.
The woman who used to
   date the drummer
   from Phish
Katie B.
M.K.
Mark K.
Jen S.
Leilani
Gavin McI.
The incarcerated
   cartoonists I stopped
   corresponding with
Felix G.
Stacey O.
Kiana K.
Laurie D.
Frank S.
The security guard I
   threw Skittles at
   in 1991
Julia W.
Ariola McS.
Cat G.
Cody G.
Dean D.
Sarah W.
The man in the Jeep at
   the intersection of
   King & University
   in 2003
Pawl K.

James R.
Emily D.
Emily S.
Iris D.
Jess A.
Lillian F.
Mackenzie
Myrtle vonD.
Pat B.
Sarah P.
Stefan J.
Suzie F.
Zane F.
Lani
Mindy
Rob B.
Jamie M.
The woman I insisted
   on "fist-bumping"
   at a party in Jackson
   Heights in 2010
Every little-league
   coach & teammate
The attendees of the
   2001 PAZ conference
Genevieve W.
Mollie W.
Matty & the Midden
The woman who sat
   next to me at
   Powell's in 1993
Minette L.
The bouncer at
   Magoo's in 1998
Jonah R.
Al & Francis
Chuck
Krazy Bill
Jacie J.
Mom
Dad
The sovereign nation
   of Hawai'i

and

Henry Henkel

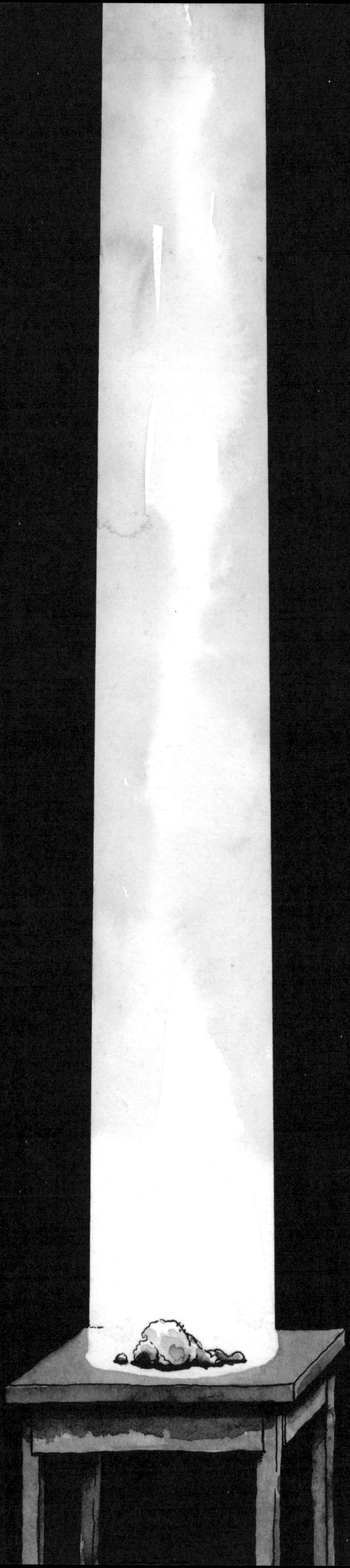

Gabby Schulz (aka Ken Dahl) is the author of Monsters, Weather, and Welcome to the Dahlhouse.

He was born and raised in Honolulu, Hawaii.